Lee Sturgeon - Day
7765 Southcliff Drive
Fair Oaks, CA 95628

Dear Thomas Moore,

First, I'd like to thank you for your writings, many of which I've read, and these with the greatest pleasure. This shift of perspective (and practice) was certainly due in the field of psychotherapy and I'm grateful that you could articulate it so concretely and humanly. I've recommended Care of the Soul to many, and will continue to do so.

Next, I'm enclosing a copy of my own book - A Slice Of Life. While I know you know of anthroposophy, I did not know how aware you might be of the medical/therapeutic work. In describing my own experiences of healing (particularly at the Lukas Klinic -Chs 20-22), I feel I am describing "Care" in Ficino's understanding and practice, and hoped you might be glad to learn something of this (and in a pretty swiftly readable form!)

Then, when reading your Planets Within, I kept asking myself if you knew of the work of astrosophy (also developed out of anthroposophy). Among others, William Bento (a friend and sometime colleague of Robert Sardello, who also wrote an introduction to my book), does - in my view - extraordinarily

A SLICE OF LIFE

A SLICE OF LIFE

A personal story of
healing through cancer

by
Lee Sturgeon-Day

LIFE&WAYS

Royal Oak, Michigan

Publisher's Cataloging in Publication Data
Sturgeon-Day, Lee, 1941 –

      A slice of life: a personal story of healing through
      cancer / by Lee Sturgeon-Day
           p.   cm.
      1. Cancer—Breast.   2. Cancer — Alternative therapy.
           3. Cancer —Personal narratives.
I. Title
RC280.B8   1991   616.99A   91-60306
ISBN 0-9628760-0-3

Printed in the United States of America

For my Blood and
Spirit Family

Acknowledgments

So many people have brought their particular gifts and talents to the making of this book: artistic, practical and, above all, their inner qualities of patience, enthusiasm and caring, that I cannot mention them all by name. Yet I know now that this is not "my" book, but "our" book. What began as an individual initiative has become a group creation. And I thereby owe to all who have participated in this modest venture the realization of a long-held vision – that of people working together creatively towards a common goal. I thank them all.

CONTENTS

Acknowledgements vi

Foreword by Robert Sardello ix

Preface xi

1. Diagnosis 3

2. Tree 9

3. Decisions 13

4. Mistletoe 19

5. Hospital 25

6. First Steps 31

7. Voices 36

8. Doctors 39

9. Diet 47

10. Fever Baths & Other Delights 56

11. Organ Rubs 63

12. Spiritual Healing 67

13. Progress? 71

14. Explorer 79

15. Questions 84

16. Winter 89

17. No-Man's Land 94

18. Into The Dark 99

19. Spring 102

20. Mecca 109

21. Healing Days 121

22. Partings 129

23. Return 140

References 146

Remembrance 148

Foreword

I am quite convinced after reading this book that disease constitutes a spiritual path for the present time, a threshold experience which can make us conscious of our life destiny. I believe it would be a mistake to read Lee Sturgeon-Day's story of her struggle with cancer as simply a personal story of one individual's fight against disease. As with all works of true imagination, we are taken into something universal. Through the many images of this story, disease is taken into the soul where it is possible to see the transformation of a life and the birth of unselfish love. Lee has asked the Grail question – "What ails thee?" – of herself, and takes us through a journey toward self-knowledge united with true feelings of the heart. Then, through this telling, we are invited to see a new vision – spiritual life is no longer found in the secluded monastic life, nor the temple, nor the church, but through the way in which we take up our deepest afflictions.

Robert Sardello
January 1991

Dr. Sardello is a psychotherapist, author of *Facing The World With Soul*, and co-director of the Dallas Institute of Humanities & Culture.

Preface

On National Cancer Day, November 1990, this book was accepted for publication and I had my annual mammogram showing "*absolutely no evidence*" of a recurrence of the breast cancer diagnosed three years before. I can count myself one of the "lucky" ones. Since writing this book several friends have died of cancer. Some chose conventional treatments, others a variety of alternatives. Some used both. The same is true for others who are still alive.

Reflecting on this, I feel our living and dying is, ultimately, a matter of destiny. By "destiny", I mean that our paths are guided by a deeper wisdom both within ourselves and within the universe than we may ever glimpse with our everyday consciousness. The true causes, meaning and purpose of what befalls us or where our acts may carry us may remain a mystery. Yet I believe that nothing we think, or feel, or do is lost; that the choices we make, the way we and those around us respond to the crisis of illness and, for many, the heroic struggle to overcome, or indeed endure it, not only shapes us, but leaves its imprint on the world. Something can always be healed through encountering an illness. And, for those who die, it may well be a victory, not a defeat.

This book has described a little of my own journey. I call it "healing *through* cancer" because, without the cancer I would not have learned, experienced, perhaps grown as I did. For each of us the journey – inwardly and outwardly – will be unique. Yet, here and there, our paths may cross, we may look out over a similar landscape, and perhaps draw comfort and courage from the fact that we do not travel alone. I wrote this book to share some of the resources for healing, particularly anthroposophic medicine and therapies, that others might like to know about. I wrote it in gratitude to all who supported me through this time. And I wrote it for all travellers and their companions on the journey towards healing – ourselves, others, and the earth we inhabit – in which I believe we are all engaged.

Lee Sturgeon-Day
December 1990.

"As every flower fades and as all youth
Departs, so life at every stage,
So every virtue, so our grasp of truth
Blooms in its day and may not last forever.
Since life may summon us at every age
Be ready, heart, for parting, new endeavor.
Be ready bravely and without remorse
To find new light that old ties cannot give.
In all beginnings dwells a magic force
For guarding us and helping us to live . . .

Even the hour of our death may send
Us speeding on to fresh and newer spaces . . ."

           – from Stages, Hermann Hesse.

"Only with friends can a man have hope
in this sacred adventure we call life."

– Prison Journals of a Priest Revolutionary, Philip Berrigan.

Chapter 1

DIAGNOSIS

"Doctors, by God; washing their hands, looking out windows, fiddling with dreadful things while you are stretched out on a table or half undressed on a chair." He finished in a voice that wailed with weakness and fury. "I'm glad I didn't finish medical school. I wouldn't have it on my soul nor conscience."
— Clock Without Hands, Carson McCullors.

The sisterhood of women has broken. Maybe it's just suspended. We sit in a row in our skimpy gowns. On video, the immaculate woman doctor is intoning, for the fifth time, the procedure for a breast exam. Just that note of severity that implies, should we fail to follow her instructions, we will have no-one but ourselves to blame. We are silent. We do not catch each other's eye. Now, on screen, the model appears, equally elegant and assured, though naked to the waist, her head robed in a yellow towel. She moves before a mirror languorously, handling her breasts. She spreads herself upon a bed to handle them some more. Quite an auto-erotic display; fun and games; while the doctor's voice offstage gives further directives in the manner of a British governess. How delicious, the model conveys, to feel one's breasts' soft contours – lump-free, naturally. Mine are shrivelled, bruised by the mammogram machine, and quite some prodding and poking by an examining nurse. Maybe I'll go home, touch and caress them myself.

Are others thinking the same? What *is* going on in this little company? Why don't we speak? Turn our heads? Howl, cling? We flip through pamphlets with averted eyes. One braves the coffee machine. Coffee is bad for us, but that's all they serve here. "They also serve who only stand and wait." So we wait, mutely, for the results.

One by one we are summoned. There are two ways to go: back to the locker room to dress, scuttle out into the fresh air; or inward, to the sanctum, where the high priests wait, polishing their words. No scalpels yet; just the initial incisions into the fabric of our lives.

When my turn comes, I am called inward for the first time in three years. I watch my body move down the corridor, my mouth making polite small talk. Not a piece out of place; British to the last ditch. "Never show feelings, girls. Moral fibre is what we develop here." Gristle that holds the flesh together, that tightens mind and heart. No, I do not fall apart at the first whiff of danger, not outwardly, though my heart has set up some outreach program somewhere between my ears and jaw. But here we are, in a small dark chamber, with the altar covered in buff files and, flaring against the backcloth, a vast lighted screen upon which, hugely magnified, is the esoteric script of the interior of my breasts.

Here," says the doctor. "This is what I'm concerned about." I give it my best attention, but I can't see a thing. It all looks the same to me; a uniform mass of grey and white squiggles I'm too illiterate to read. Even when the doctor circles a spot with her felt-tipped pen, it seems a random choice on her part. How do I know these are my breasts anyway?

"I'd recommend a biopsy of this spot."

"Oh-er, well, if you say so."

"It would be wise." Oh, let us be wise. Let us defer to those who do know about such things.

"Do you know a surgeon? Have you anyone to go to?"

"Well, I have a friend. She had a biopsy once . . ."

"Of course, if you know someone. Otherwise I'd recommend a very good woman surgeon here. You'd like her." Yes, a woman. One I might like too. Let us defer again.

"Well – if you recommend her –"

"I do. She's excellent." Before I can change my mind, the doctor makes the appointment, there and then, on the telephone, for the following week.

"Good luck," she says, as I gather my robe around me, and prepare to depart. "Let me know how it goes."

In the parking lot my legs give way. I feel the tremors run down my thighs. "Can you drive home?" I ask of myself, as I clamber like an octogenarian into my car. "Yes," a distant voice replies. Where are the women now? Where are the voices to comfort, the arms to uplift? Come on, Lee, you're a woman yourself. Take deep breaths; summon something, someone to your aid. It is a man who comes. John Davy, who died of the disease I am suspected of. So – he is dead. Want a bet? He's here now, green in my memory, in the medical complex parking lot. As I remember him, feel the warmth of his presence, the trembling subsides. I begin to breathe evenly. I begin to smile. So, all set to go, foot on the accelerator, first stage of this new journey, one mile at a time.

*   *   *

It's a bleak grey morning when Lulu and I drive downtown. Phase 2: Biopsy. I wonder how many thousands of women the world over are doing, or having done to them, this today. How many surgeons dressing, grabbing cups of coffee, driving crowded freeways, sitting in subways, or maybe jogging down rough country lanes, to be there in time to sharpen their knives? I hope the other women have company as fine as mine. Lulu's name, in another lifephase, was Lulu Darling. It's apt for this lovely, loyal friend and ally on this odyssey.

"I have to stop for gas," she says, as we exit on Warren towards the concrete and brick citadel of Detroit's Medical Center.

"Sure."

"God, my knees are shaking. Do you mind if I have a cigarette?"

"Let's share one. It's a bit late to worry about those!"

"We don't know yet," Lulu reminds me. "We must be hopeful."

"Yes." Yes, we must be hopeful. Yet I honestly don't know what I am hoping for. Mainly to get through the next hours creditably, and enjoy a good lunch afterwards. I imagine the cooks at the Traffic Jam and Snug, busy too with their knives, and decide to hope for vegetable soup and parmezan bread and, yes, for a good strong mug of tea – the British ritual cure for all life's little disturbances.

At 8:30 a.m. we arrive. Lulu waits in the waiting room. I am ushered into the sanctum and, fairly quickly, having stripped to the waist, am impaled upon the mammogram machine. As many well know, this is a vice that imprisons your breasts, (pretty painfully in the case of small ones, there being so little to imprison and always the danger of catching something else as well,) and you stand, muttering prayerful incantations while the X-ray lady retires to buzz the buzzer that signals the taking of the X-ray. My chief prayer is that my legs won't give out, for the vice certainly won't, and will hang on to my breast wherever the rest of me goes to.

Today, there are some differences. Firstly, to my great relief, I can sit on a chair. But – I am warned – I'll be in the vice for around half an hour. It is also a vice with a difference, for it has holes in it. And through one of these holes a needle will be inserted into my breast.

"Well, it's more like a screw, isn't it," says the doctor, to whom I presume is a medical student. "Can you feel how it screws into the fat?"

Yes, I can. It *is* more like a screw.

"Oh dear, you do bleed easily." Someone goes to get some Kleenex as I'm obviously spoiling the machine. We can't have a messy machine for the next customer. I can see nothing of this, because my own head is screwed over an angle of chrome, and I obviously don't dare move. I'll see the bloodshed later.

"It's a very long needle," says the doctor. "We'll cut it off later. Now, let's see if we got the right place." So the buzzer buzzes, and we all wait while the X-ray is developed, making chatty conversation to take our minds off things.

Happily, we did get the right place – the "area", as it will henceforth be called. So I am unleashed somewhat gingerly, so the needle doesn't drop out and we have to begin all over again. It's a lovely job, I gather; absolutely hit the target. But, oh dear, there is rather a lot of blood. My breast continues to drip on to the machine, and people take turns mopping. Then a rinky-dink paper cup is put over the needle and an equally rinky-dink paper gown over me. I am returned to the waiting room. Here Lulu and I make further conversation. The doctor joins us for a while, and gives me my file. Now we have the "area" and the "case" all tidily together.

Eventually, a young hospital orderly appears with a wheelchair. I hop in with

Lulu's bags, and we set off on a mile or so journey underground to another hospital.

Here it is pretty cold. I ask a nurse for surgical socks. There aren't any. I ask for a couple of thick blankets. There aren't any. But I do get one thin one. (It will be a triumphant day for medical science when it is discovered that patients tend to feel the cold. I won't even bother to mention yet that the cancer patient feels particularly cold and anyone even remotely suspected of this disease should be kept warmer than anyone else.)

I now strip below the waist too and sit, feeling fairly undignified, reading a book while the nurse shuffles her notes. Lulu is, yet again, in the waiting room, this time filled with sickly green, mauve and orange chairs, clearly chosen by some sadist who believes the weak and their consorts should be expunged from the earth's surface with all possible speed.

After about half an hour reading, I'm led into the operating room. This is colder still. I mount the table, and the nurse begins to prepare me for this initiation, robing me in blue cloths, (except for the "area", which is ceremonially painted several coats of a brownish yellow liquid. She carefully traces round the needle, from which the paper cup has now been removed.) The blue cloths offset the tawny gold of my breast, but I'm really too cold to appreciate the artistry.

After another wait, my surgeon arrives; lovely and cheerful, apologizing – and who can blame her – for her own icy hands. Dr. Pamela Benitez is a violinist, and writes poetry, as well as carving people up. She tells me she chose surgery, so she could do something artistic in the medical field.
"So were you the Amazon in another life, or was I?" I ask, as she selects her blade. It is all so ritualistic, and this is the most obvious ritual to identify with.
"Well, I certainly was," she replies.
"Perhaps that makes two of us?" I do wonder if Amazons cut off their own breasts, or got a friend to do it for them, and how I might discover this. But the image is adequate for now, and I lie thinking what in my remote past might have led me to this moment, and also assuring myself that certainly in many other lives far worse things have befallen me. Today, thanks to western advances, I am locally anesthetized. And thanks to Dr. Benitez, the cloths are artfully suspended around my head, leaving me in a dim blue cave, so that I don't actually have to watch what's happening. I can, of course, hear. There's lots of snip-snipping of tough fiber. I think of the annual pruning of my garden shrubs: rosebush, clematis, forsythia. I feel I do need pruning too. I half wish Dr. Benitez could – artistically of course – divest me of all the woody, fibrous branches in both breasts and I could make a fresh start with delicious new, tender, healthy growth. But she does what we've agreed she'll do, and removes part of the "area". This is then put in something – I presume – and carted back to the other doctor for a further X-ray to make sure it's the right place. I imagine another orderly, hot-footing it Olympically down the tunnels, carrying this piece of flesh, and hope he doesn't drop it to be mangled in to the concrete by the next oncoming patient's wheelchair.

The waiting part is not thrilling. The anesthetic begins to wear off. I am rather sickeningly aware that my breast is wide open, and it will feel much safer and better when Dr. Benitez can stitch it closed again. Eventually this phase is reached. Several Bandaids are applied, and I'm ready to go. No hot tea! I just totter out, dress, and go in search of Lulu. We rush to the Traffic Jam & Snug for big bowls of barley soup, which we both sorely need. The whole enterprise has taken around three hours.

The results take longer; a time of suspense. In fact, I feel utterly suspended; my legs heavy and inert as if hanging over a surface I cannot yet reach or touch. It is an effort to carry out garbage, get to and from the grocery store. The presence of an event I know is coming to meet me, but whose shape is still veiled, keeps me transfixed, paralyzed, through the next three days. I think of little else.

I wonder why "they" take so much time? Is there a pile-up in the labs, like a sorting room after a postal strike? What do they do to the "received fresh tissue" before they know beyond a shadow of a doubt? I think of white-coated experts bent over myriad lumps of flesh. What a life! Do they ever mix them up? I can make no plans myself. Any based on having cancer might bring a self-fulfilling prophecy. Yet any that leave me cancer-free could be an utter waste of time. How I hate waiting for anything, too; good, or bad.

When Lulu and I go back to the hospital for Dr. Benitez to deliver the verdict, we have covered the bases of both alternatives: "to have" or "not to have". And, having sat interminably on the orange and lime-green chairs, we are somewhat undone by a third, unconsidered option, which is that the results have still not come through. I trail miserably home, wondering if I can stand a whole weekend of uncertainty.

By two o-clock, I decide I can't. I break with my British traditions: "Don't make a fuss"; "Join the queue," and start calling the hospital every hour, telling them to page Dr. Benitez wherever she is; slicing up bodies, or sitting in the cafeteria, I don't care which. And this forcefulness pays off. At 5:30 p.m., just before she leaves for the weekend, I hear her voice, matter of factly telling me that I do have a malignancy, entitled "intraductal carcinoma", and suggesting we meet on Monday to discuss my options. I get myself somewhat shakily to the dinner table and dole out chicken and mashed potatoes to Lulu and Adam, my nine-year old son, while my own stomach rises in protest and my own mouth continues to make dinner conversation with them both.

As Lulu is putting on her coat to leave, I mutter my news. She looks at me long and hard.

"Do you want me to stay?"

"No. No, I'll be all right." We hold each other's gaze, for I owe her nothing less than the truth.

"Do you want a hug?"

"Yes. Yes, please." She folds me tightly in her arms for a long, long time. I'd

like to stay there forever, like a child being comforted from a bad dream. Though it isn't a dream, I do feel comforted, and begin to breathe evenly again. As we pull apart, she says:
"I'll call you tomorrow, when Adam's not around."
"Thanks." With a last warm squeeze, she lets me go.
"I love you," she says.
"I love you too."
I put Adam to bed. This isn't the time to tell him anything. Our evening ritual of stories, cuddles, prayers, is full of a haunting tenderness. I creep in later, and watch him sleeping, his small, untroubled face snuggled beside his large family of furry animals. He is *my* family. With a deep sigh I turn to my own bed.

Very slowly the fact washes over me. I have cancer. And, in its wake, follows a curious calm. Michael Crichton captures such a moment delightfully, in his autobiography, *Travels*, which I read later this year.

"We can all work ourselves into a hysterical panic over possibilities we won't look at. What if I have cancer? What if my job is at risk? What if my kids are on drugs? What if I'm getting bald? What if there's an elephant outside my tent?
And that hysteria goes away the instant we are willing to hear the answer. Even if that answer is what we feared all along. Yes, you have cancer. Yes, your kids are on drugs. Yes, there's an elephant outside your tent."

The elephant standing so solidly outside my tent is far less threatening than the distant sound of one stampeding through the jungle on its way to attack. I even chuckle to myself: "at least there's one thing less to be afraid of; getting cancer. I've got it now!" And I recall similar moments when the terror of awaiting a "worst thing" – the end of a love affair, some humiliating failure – is replaced, at least temporarily, by an almost mystical calm when the event actually, factually occurs.
But the night is long, and not wholly calm. One deep terror comes, that I know will pursue me again and again. "What about Adam, if I die?" It surfaces like some ancient, malevolent seamonster, rising from those dark depths in which lie all our losses, loves and wounds, all my ferocious, protective instincts towards this child of my flesh, this being of my heart. I will not surrender our connection lightly. Nor can I bear to think of it fracturing now. Indeed, each time this monster rises and plunges towards me, I back off hastily. Then, to my surprise, another creature, perched on my shoulder, seems to murmur: "You'll still be alive tomorrow. Both you and he." As if to reassure myself, I tiptoe to his room again; bend over his sprawled, slight form in red pyjamas, tenderly touch his tousled hair. Yes, we have tomorrow, and surely many more. "One day at a time," I tell myself, as I am to do so often. "And you do not know what tomorrow will bring." The monster retreats as I return to my own room and, yes, sleep like a child myself.

Chapter 2

TREE

"Someday someone will isolate the frequency of love and build a machine to transmit it. Calling it Smith's Healing Rays, they will charge it to beam at our injured parts. And we may forget it was ours all the time. But for now, we call it Tree."
                                              – Tree. Deena Metzger.

At 11 a.m. the following day the telephone rings.
"Lee, it's Catherine."
"Catherine! Why aren't you asleep?" It is three hours earlier in Boulder, Colorado and I know how much my friend relishes a lie-in after a heavy week's work.
"I got your news. I didn't want to miss you."
"How did you get my news?" I feel this morning, even after a largish cup of coffee, that I've hardly got it myself.
"Paula called."
"But I haven't seen Paula in three months!"
"She called Irene yesterday, because she felt something was wrong with one of us. Irene told her about you. So she called me right away."
        How can this be? I had forgotten Irene's call to me. Yet Paula, my friend and lawyer, whom I sadly see so seldom, was urged towards me; an uncanny pull from the web of connection that binds so many of us and which, in her turn, she tugs on to bring the clear voice of Catherine, full of concern, love, hope; offering over the miles a hand to hold, a source of sustaining energy. So this is what "tomorrow" brings. And that is not the whole of it.
        In the hours and days that follow, the network surfaces; first here in Detroit, then further afield: Arizona, New York, England, Wales, Holland, Canada; voices travelling across oceans, letters and cards. Those close to home pay visits, ask what I need, what they can do.
        Cynthia is one of the first. She lives next door. It is from her that I get my next hug. I cry in her arms. I've never done that before and wonder why I have deprived myself of such warm and ready comfort. I've certainly had plenty to cry about in the years we've known each other. It is she, too, who is ready to step in with practical help. When others, myself included, may be straining our emotions on behalf of someone in distress, Cynthia will probably have cleaned their house and baked a year's supply of chocolate cake! So here she is now, already

9

wondering if she could get across to Canada to bring back supplies of healthy vegetables to build my vitality before the surgery. I don't even need to ask if she'll take care of Adam. She offers to do so, anytime and anyplace.

Mary-Jo is instantly beside me, with Rob's sustaining presence waiting in the wings. She has struggled for years with fragile health and is full of wise advice and sympathy. Vibrant with warmth and humor, even when grappling with painful allergic reactions to food or environmental pollutants, she images the fruits of this struggle in her sensitivity to others embarking on a healing course. Her sensitivities are probably what make her such an excellent remedial teacher too, for our curses are our gifts as well. I know that her support and counsel will carry me through the many changes I will be trying to make.

Other members of my immediate group are equally quick to respond; Karen and Paul, Francina and Howard, Lora, Dori, Conrad, Susanne, and many more. Here they come – this steadfast company. I do not travel alone!

A few days later my parents call in response to my letter. I could not at first face the telephone. It is them I most hate telling, for who can restrain an anguished concern for their own child – even if that child is almost a relic herself! If Adam's smallest hurts and sorrows twist in my gut, how must this touch them?

"Don't worry about money," my stepfather says gruffly. "Just let us know what you need." Typical. Love in action. We may never talk about this thing, yet I think he would return from the hereafter to *do* something for me.

My mother offers to come for a couple of weeks after my surgery. I am grateful and glad; for time with this kindred spirit, who is also the woman from whose womb I was reluctantly dragged over forty years ago. She has bandaged my knees, administered Friar's Balsam Inhalers, brought me through mumps and measles, even miscarriages, with her brisk efficiency. Now I need her, not just for the efficiency! I need her wise mind, her support of my choices, however bizarre, the strength of her often hidden heart. I need her for Adam too – perhaps the most greatly loved constant in his life – at a time when I may be threateningly in flux. This is time for the truly familiar, for both of us – before moving into strange and frightening territory. And who can be more familiar than one's own family? The struggles, the frequent collision of differing personalities, the years both good and bad, have forged enduring bonds. By the time my brother and sister have also responded, each in their distinctive ways, I feel like a well-equipped hiker, ready to face blizzards and earthquakes which may destroy me but which will not find me lacking food, a warm bedroll and all my emergency supplies.

But what of others – my spirit kin? I expect Jane to care. Archie, her son, my godson, died of an inoperable brain tumor, but not before teaching us all we ever need to know and bringing those who knew him abidingly close. But I do not expect her voice on the telephone, beaming across the Atlantic within hours of getting my news. Nor Francie's – the same day. From east and west of the British Isles. Their familiar English inflections, particular warmth, dry wit, (that perhaps few Americans can really understand,) make me suddenly homesick for the penetrating cold and damp of an English November, full of drizzle and acrid, rotting smells. I am almost tempted to get on a plane – which of course they encourage me to do.

Nor am I expecting Mike's call. Though a family friend, I don't think I've seen him in fifteen years.

"I was bloody angry with your brother," he booms. "He hinted that there was something up with you, but was so super-secretive I had to get your number from your mother in the end." Did I respond with such fervor when Mike lived through his own ordeal that cost him the sight in one eye?

What is happening, too, when I go to make my meager purchases at Cameron Meats, the Amish store in Ferndale that I've recently discovered and apologize to the proprietor that I may be turning vegetarian? When reaching for my packages, he does not pass them to me, but takes my hands in his large workworn ones. "Cold," he comments. "Can't have that, can we?" He proceeds to warm my chilly fingers, not to mention what he's doing to my heart. He does not know I'm sick. Is it obvious? No, I think some stupid barrier in me has broken to allow this meeting, but it still astonishes.

I probably shed more tears in the following week than in the preceding decade. They are tears of joy; not without pain, as true joy seldom is, for I feel humbled and vulnerable to this loving energy. At times I really cannot believe it and wonder if there's been a big mistake; that it is really meant for someone else. Once in Bangkok, a hotel clerk thrust an immense bunch of orchids into my arms, thinking I was Shirley MacLaine, and I had to return it when he discovered his error. Perhaps I'll wake up one morning and find I'll have to return all this care and concern.

Sometimes – I confess – it might feel easier to do so, for I do not know if I can bear it and all it implies for me, my life.

"I was so angry," says Marjorie. "I prayed, but I was so angry with God. I said: '"You can't take her from us'".

Sheila writes: "You must get better. You must be healed. This is a COM-MAND!"

Ouch! My most secret places of self-abuse and self-denial are grievously assaulted. Wounds that have not seen the light of day for years re-open glaringly. "We need you." "You are important." Why, or for what, I do not know. Once I try asking, hoping for some image to shield me from the abyss, a name to give form to the chaos I feel is me and also so often feel might better be simply dissolved, return to whence it came. But no-one really answers me. And that's right too. We are all needed. Each one equally. And labels, reasons, more often than not, are crutches, weapons to defend ourselves against the terrifying fact of our uniqueness and the imperious call again and again to grow, become more and more the person we were meant to be. This call weakens my own defences. I feel the crusted layers begin to crumble with each loving invasion. It hurts, and I am afraid.

"Now I wait in terror for the spring
That comes like blood to unbound feet . . ."

So my friend, the poet and writer Judith Thurman, wrote twenty years ago, yet I never felt it as I do now. And when I am not in shock, or tears, or moved by simple gratitude, there's a growing sense of wonder and awe that such a potential exists – for all of us.

"The thing is," says Cammie, "that it's a real power that we don't use. At least I don't, except in an emergency." She tells me of her own thoughts sent silently across the continent to another friend in crisis, who reported – though ignorant of this – how healed she felt: "As if you were actually helping me."

"I know. We believe it. We preach it. We have evidence. Yet we seldom use it – and we're surprised when it works." For, whatever else is happening in me, I am clearly aware that since the network became active I've felt little fear of the cancer, or of the impending surgery.

Cammie and I look at each other, perplexed; each maybe travelling inward to some place in the heart that feels shame, and a kind of wondering hope that we might, just might be able to evolve. . .touch, care, heal. . . .

"I guess that's why we need these emergencies," I say ruefully. "If we did this every day for each other, as a matter of course. . ."

Yes why don't we? Standing with Cammie on my front doorstep in the thin November sunshine, I wonder why – at least why I do not. Perhaps this is one of the first deep lessons the cancer begins to teach me – that we are nothing without each other, and have more powers together than we know. When another friend gives me *The Bone People*, I read Keri Hume's words for it.

"They were nothing more than people, by themselves. Even paired, any pairing, they would have been nothing more than people by themselves. But all together, they have become the heart and muscles and mind of something perilous and new, something strange and growing and great. Together, all together, they are the instruments of change."

So I feel us gathering; my being gathered by these people; steadied for the leap into whatever perils await us all.

Chapter 3

DECISIONS

"If there were a devil he would not be the one who decided against God, but he that in all eternity did not decide."
— I and Thou, Martin Buber.

It's not just a matter of sitting around soaking up love and concern. I have decisions to make. I marvel at the energy we find in crisis that may be sorely lacking at other times. In my case, it's probably the influence of the British folk soul. Though we seldom complain, or are moved to passionate action, give us a crisis: a war, a disaster, and we are roused like no other beast. We thrive in adversity. In these first days I feel vigorous and definite; my fighting spirit coming to the fore. One choice – to follow an alternative treatment after surgery – is quickly made. Now for the surgery itself.

Pamela Benitez tells me I should choose between a modified mastectomy and a lumpectomy.

"A quandrantectomy, actually," she explains. "I'd remove about a quarter of your breast and a section of lymph nodes to see if it's spread."

Neither sound particularly nice to me, but a quarter has the edge over the whole for me. I have a hard time letting go of anything. Small though my breasts are, I'm still curiously attached to them.

I'm pretty certain Pamela told me that the recommended package is to follow a quandratectomy with radiation. But I didn't hear this. The pamphlet she was required by law to give me (and I was probably required by law to read) confirms this fact. At the time I barely glanced at it. My vision blurred at the sight of anatomical diagrams, incomprehensible jargon, or horrid words that were only too clear: 'malignant', 'tumor', 'quick-spreading', etc. Cancer, I reflected, snapping the book shut rapidly, is the only disease described in the language of evil. I'll deal with that one later. Enough is more than enough.

I tell Pamela I want to wait two weeks for surgery. I need time to rake my leaves and put my garden to bed. My voice sounds defiant. It surprises me. And so does her reply.

"Good idea. You just let me know what day suits you best."

I relax, feeling instantly affirmed. Pamela has helped me over a reef of panic, too: panic that the cancer would kill me before I got to the operating table. She would hardly do herself out of a job, would she? I think the lay person, particularly of my generation, has absorbed this frightening notion – cancer is a killer – and I had not yet read the many stories of cures. Even my mother, calling again from England, is momentarily swayed.

"But, darling! Putting it off just for your leaves?"

"Yes." Yes, this small choice was an infinitely important one. Not merely practical – for I could hardly rake leaves after surgery – but a psychological victory. Though I have plenty of fears, I will not act out of them. Pamela is the first doctor who awakens this resolution. Emboldened by her support, I tell her I shall certainly be following surgery with a little known treatment – mistletoe therapy.

"Sounds intriguing," she says. "I'd like to hear more about it, if you have any literature."

Another threshold is crossed. How often am I to hear in the coming months that it is pointless, even destructive, to tell conventional physicians about alternatives. I was to discover how tough it could be at times. But the fates guided me again and again to certain professionals who were open, accepting and deeply encouraging, and to whom I was and am still intensely grateful. It is their courage, I think: the courage to stand within a certain framework and still imagine it does not hold all the answers, that helped me find my own courage to fumble my way through so many conflicting opinions to what I believed was right for me. I leave Pamela's office pretty buoyed up.

*   *   *

The alternative treatment I had mentioned to her stems from what is called "anthroposophically-extended" medicine. Though widely practised in many countries, it is barely known here, so I will attempt a thumbnail sketch of it.

This medical approach was developed in the early part of this century by the Austrian philosopher and scientist, Rudolf Steiner, together with physicians who sought to broaden the narrow perspective of a purely physical approach to illness which characterizes western medicine today.

Dr. Steiner's insights have been carried into many fields: agriculture, the arts, economic and social initiatives and, notably, Waldorf education – one of the largest alternative school movements in the world. His system of thought and practice is known as Anthroposophy (wisdom of man), or Spiritual Science. As the latter title implies, it is an exacting training in thought and perception, as disciplined as that of the natural sciences, yet one whereby faculties can be developed that enable a person to perceive the spiritual forces active within the material world. Many of Dr. Steiner's own insights have been verified in recent years by scientists themselves, who have extended their own frontiers of knowledge since his time. (He died in 1925.)

I had been a student of Anthroposophy for many years, drawn to a spiritual world-view whose truths – while immensely complex and challenging – could work so practically and transformatively into daily life. Those I met, for whom Anthroposophy was the basis of their lives and work, and the many initiatives that showed the creative effect of such perceptions and insights in practice, continually inspired and impressed me. Thus began what one fellow traveller has described as "the most exciting, eccentric, fulfilling, frustrating, and common-sensible journey I have ever taken." One which led me, among other inner and outer paths, to seek help from anthroposophic doctors when I needed it.

The medical work illustrates most clearly the combination of scientific exactitude and what I would call an artistic, even religious, consciousness. As one doctor comments: "I see anthroposophical medicine at a turning point where we cannot necessarily reject what has been developed by modern medicine but we must see that in its specialization it's grown much too one-sided. It doesn't see the whole picture. We are trying to add a wider image of the interplay of physical and spiritual factors in health and illness, in addition to considering the effects of environment, heredity, individual destiny. . . ."

In one of the best introductions to this extremely complex system, *Anthroposophic Medicine Today*, the author, Richard Leviton states that it may be the therapeutic approach of the 21st century, combining scientific precision with spiritual depth – hopefully in one competent physician! So, although it does restore some of the lost elements of healing, and uses terminology that we may more readily associate with religious systems, it is not a return to the past, but is strongly committed to development into the future.

An anthroposophical doctor is a qualified MD. (This need not be so of someone practising homeopathy, with which anthroposophical medicine has much in common.) Beyond a full conventional training, an anthroposophical physician follows a rigorous discipline, a path of both inner and outer development, designed to lead him or her to a deep perception of the forces active in the human being and in nature, (from which the medications will be derived.) These forces, though invisible to most of us, may still be seen in their effects within the physical organism, so that before one is able to perceive them "spiritually" one can observe and understand their workings in material phenomena.

One essential model for grasping something of this approach is Steiner's "Fourfold image of man". (There are other models which complement and broaden this.) The human being is seen as being composed of three mutually interpenetrating "bodies" or "sheaths", in which the Ego – the unique individuality – incarnates and works. These are respectively: the physical body, which we have in common with the mineral world; the etheric, or life-body, which continually creates, repairs and maintains the physical body as a plant is upheld throughout its life; and the astral body, the bearer of thoughts, feelings, impulses, and the vehicle for consciousness, which we have in common with the animal kingdom. Last, but not least, is our Ego; the core, the "I Am" of our being, which distinguishes us from the rest of creation as a unique, human individuality. (Much of its full reality remains hidden from our consciousness. In this sense it is closer to Jung's concept of the Self; the archetype that underlies and shapes our destiny, than the everyday ego of his and others' psychologies.)

Each of these aspects of the human being has a specific connection with certain organs and body systems, and each functions according to distinctly different laws. One sees a reflection of the working of these forces in the physical body itself. For example, the astral body's chief sphere of action is the nerve-sense system, the physiological basis for the Ego is the blood. While the etheric body is continually replenishing the whole, (the immune-system, *par excellence*,) through the lymphatic and glandular systems, the astral body consumes the vitality of the etheric in the service of consciousness. The Ego contains not only the spiritual forces for our potential destiny, but also the blueprint for the total organism and strives to impress its formative powers throughout these other bodies, down to the last cell.

Illness is seen as arising through some disharmony between these bodies, and quite frequently the villain is the astral body whose undisciplined activity erodes the life-bringing energies of the etheric. I think it is quite easy to imagine this. We know the part our thoughts and emotions can play in our physical state; a single sleepless night spent fretting over a problem causes havoc to our sense of wellbeing the following day. Invariably, the Ego is failing to master these bodies and penetrate their activity with its formative powers.

A doctor will be looking for the particular disharmony between these bodies which has led to the expression of a physical symptom, and then seeking to restore the equilibrium. According to the various ways in which they may have fallen out with each other, treatment can vary enormously. The doctor is as likely to discern this by the way a patient walks or talks, by the form, tone, color, gesture of the patient, as through extensive physical exams or diagnostic tests. These often only serve to confirm the picture already formed. Having been a patient on several occasions, I've always felt such a doctor "sees" me in far greater depth than a conventional physician and that is always a confirming experience rather than an intrusive one.

In seeking the appropriate remedies and therapies, a similar acute observation and imaginative perception is applied, particularly to the world of nature, from which the medications are drawn. These work on the homeopathic principle of "treating like with like". Anthroposophic medicine shares much of its pharmocopoeia with homeopathy, though it has several hundred additional remedies and there are some distinctive differences in the area of dosages. Treatment usually consists of a number of elements – medication, physical and artistic therapies, counseling; and involves the patient in a quite active participation in his or her own healing process.

My sense is that such a healer needs an artist's vision as well as scientific knowledge. If we behold a painting by Michelangelo, we will hardly appreciate and understand it if we merely analyze the pigments and chemical components of the paint he used. We will need to stand back, allow the forms and colors to affect us, perhaps to question what Michelangelo intended to convey through this physical medium. While conventional medicine spends its time analyzing components of physical substance, and restoring the canvas as best it may, an anthroposophical physician will be imagining what lies behind the physical expression of an illness and, most importantly, questioning how to bring the work of art that is every human being – a work in an ongoing process of creation – into a more perfect expression.

This sense of the human being in a continual creative development is very important to me. I already accepted that my cancer was a final expression in my body of a long process of dis-ease in body, soul and spirit, that had been proceeding for many years before attaining a physical form. The lumps and bumps were a cry for help, a cry for change. I also saw it as a challenge, (one I would gladly do without in these first days, but a challenge nonetheless.) And if I survived, I hoped to get "better" in the sense of being "better" than I was before. Though I quaked at the thought of dying, and prayed some voice from heaven would quickly assure me I would not, I wanted to "make something" of this illness, or allow it to "make something" of me; to bring me to a greater wholeness, a deeper sense of myself and the world.

And this is where anthroposophical medicine had to be my path. Its goal is not simply to re-establish some lost harmony, restore the *status quo*, but to encourage and impel the patient to new levels of awareness and action. If we do not develop, the illness is wasted. One doctor I knew, once hinted darkly that we might even get a worse one if we failed to avail ourselves of the opportunity provided by the first.

Development is also emphatically not seen only in the context of a surviving life. We may be healed in some much more significant way, even though we die. That vision was tremendously important to me. I guessed I would probably lose it again and again, so I knew I would need people around me who would nudge me awake, remind me of this essential truth.

Anthroposophic medicine has a great deal to offer the cancer patient; several unique perceptions of this illness, and distinctive treatments which have been widely used with marked success over the past few decades. I knew a little about this. Friends brought me books and articles and I began to get a rough picture that I knew I'd be filling in as the weeks went by.

Cancer is termed a degenerative disease, belonging more properly to later life, as are other sclerotic, hardening diseases such as arthritis. In cancer, cells have emancipated themselves from the form and functioning of the body as a whole and do their own thing at the expense of the total organism. These cells are actually weak and confused, as well they might be, having fallen out of the body's community. Their claim to fame is their capacity to multiply at great speed, sapping the vitality of the body, often to the point of death. We all carry cancer cells, but a healthy organism deals with them effectively. It is only in the cancer patient that the body – or indeed whatever shapes and guides the body – is unable to destroy them.

Anthroposophic medicine challenges the conventional theory that organisms are made up of cells that know what they are doing, and claims rather that the shaping powers of the organism are continually battling against the tendency of the cells to proliferate indiscriminately. In cancer, these cells actually regress to an earlier state of development, slipping out of the appropriate form of the organism if the higher members of our being do not control and guide them sufficiently. So this system sees cancer arising at just those points where the formative forces are weakened, or from which they have withdrawn, leaving a space for autonomous growth.

This medical system also divides illnesses into "hot" and "cold" categories. The former, such as inflammatory illnesses and fevers, will flush through the entire system, revitalizing it in the process, filling every nook and cranny with new life. In cancer, there are critical places that are never permeated with warmth. It is therefore one of the "cold" diseases. (It is interesting that it flourishes today in a society that is quick to suppress fevers and immunize us against childhood illnesses that could keep our immune-system – always seriously depleted by the time cancer occurs – in good working order.)

Cancer, therefore, has an ideal opportunity to breed in a cold constitution; in a person who has a consistently low body temperature and seldom, if ever, runs fevers. I think this insight is, at present, unique to anthroposophic medicine. Dr. Paul Pearsall, in his recent excellent book, *Super-Immunity*, refers to hot and cold personality types, the latter being cancer-prone. Of course, if one has a cold body one may well have a cold soul – maybe it is the perennial question of which comes first, chicken or egg? But I think the perception of actual physical coldness offering a prime breeding ground for this disease is particularly valuable, because it suggests that a top priority in any treatment will be to warm us up again. This has been quite intuitively perceived by many patients who have sent their cancers into remission by jogging and other sweat-producing activities, which also increase the flow of oxygen that cancer cannot abide. And I believe the only cases of spontaneous remission have occurred where patients have run high fevers, particularly due to infections after operations which, very probably, hospital staff have been at pains to reduce, happily not always successfully.

I think we all recognize the tremendous difference we feel between the warmth we generate when we feel particularly "present" – in love, enthusiasm, anger, when we feel so fully "ourselves" – and the moments when we withdraw, retreat from our bodies, in fear or shock, and our face pales, our toes and fingers numb. Another way of describing our coldness is, then, that we are not fully incarnated within our own flesh. Our Ego is clearly not doing its job. Healing must involve warming the patient up, in any number of ways, so that the Ego, which works in the warmth of the blood, can take hold of the situation and exert its guiding influence over those areas that have fallen out into the cold.

This much I had vaguely grasped. Apart from knowing I'd have to wear woolly vests for the rest of my life, I knew only one – the most vital – ingredient of my total future therapy. This was *Viscum Album*, (mistletoe), often known by one of its brand names, *Iscador*.

Chapter 4

MISTLETOE

"We may be able to triumph over this disease in this life or we may not, but we shall always be able to bring healing in some form or other to our patients when we use this therapy."
— Illness and Healing, Dr. Rita Leroi.

I have not seen mistletoe growing since I came to live in the States, but often, playing in the woods of my childhood in Britain, we would see high up in the branches of an oak tree the dark, rounded clump of a mistletoe plant, with its pale, moony globes of berries shining between the leaves. We would gather it at Christmas, hanging it in the hallway, and no greeting was complete without kissing under it. Even in my ignorance of its meaning and significance, it seemed a special sacred plant.

It is. Since ancient times it has been attributed with healing powers. The Druids called it "all-healing" and used it in a variety of ways – to increase fecundity, treat wounds and swellings, deformed nails and, significantly, tumorous growths. It played an important part in pagan rites and sacrifices. This may be why it is banned in many Christian churches to this day. Quite recently, when archaeologists disinterred the "Lindow Man", killed around 300 BC, three grains of mistletoe pollen were discovered in his stomach. It is not known whether he took it to increase his magical powers, or to treat a stomach tumor.

It also features in Norse mythology where the sun god, Baldur, is slain by a mistletoe dart prepared by the evil Loki in a fit of rage and jealousy. All the substances of the earth had pledged not to harm Baldur, but no-one thought to extract such a promise from the mistletoe, since it barely belongs to the earth.

Why might it heal cancer? Clearly the Druids believed it did. And Rudolf Steiner restored this function to it in the early part of this century. He showed how one can observe in the plant itself both the gesture of cancer and qualities that cancer lacks and needs if those cells are to be re-educated into the proper form and function again.

Like cancer, mistletoe is a parasite. It nourishes itself from the host tree and can eventually destroy this. It ignores earthly laws, through living outside gravity and pursuing its cycles of growth and decay with no regard for the seasons. Bud and fruit can be found on the same plant at any time of the year. Cancer breaks the rules too, pursuing its own growth regardless of its environment and therefore at the expense of it.

19

The positive qualities of mistletoe are a capacity to bring light and form. The sinkers embedded in the host tree are actually green though they never see the light. The wonderfully rounded shape of a clump of mistletoe testifies to its formative powers. It generally grows on trees that live near water, shaping itself out of this fluid element. Form and light are what cancer so significantly lacks. Mistletoe introduces the possibility of restoring these elements.

Interestingly, both cancer cells and mistletoe are arrested at an earlier phase of evolution, both of the earth and of the human being. Perhaps, through their mutual interaction, both can be brought forward now. Might this redeem the killing power of mistletoe in Baldur's time? For evil is surely the wrong thing in the wrong place at the wrong time. I ponder this as I learn more about these two regressive characters.

Since Rudolf Steiner gave these indications, mistletoe has been used increasingly by a large number of physicians – particularly in Europe – for thousands of cancer patients with significantly positive results. Some use it in conjunction with drugs or radiation. This is proving more effective than the latter alone. Many are choosing it as an alternative. It is also prescribed for pre-cancerous conditions, which can be diagnosed by a "blood-crystallization" test – an interesting tool of anthroposophic medicine. Mistletoe is also beginning to show positive results with some AIDS sufferers.

Analysis of its properties – now possible with modern techniques which were not available in Steiner's time, reveal a sound basis for treating cancer. I'm no chemist! I know it has a dual function which no other treatment has. It acts cytostatically (as does chemotherapy) in destroying cancer cells. It also stimulates the immune-system, notably increasing lymphocytes which in turn attack malignant cells. It is administered by injection, usually subcutaneously, and in cycles of increasing potency.

Research and development in this field continues, under the rigorous conditions rightly imposed by the scientific community, with the notable exception that there be no blind or double-blind testing. If a patient wants mistletoe, that is what he or she will get. It is considered unethical to use duplicity where a patient's life and choices are concerned.

Getting hold of this medication here in the States is one of the first acts of will required of a patient. It is not banned by the FDA, but is still "unapproved". It must be imported from Europe, and can only be prescribed by a physician with experience of this therapy. Though I frequently groused at the effort: the time, money and energy spent in pursuing my particular therapies in this country, I also reflected that this same effort might play a part in my cure. Happily, the first step was relatively easy for me. I knew about mistletoe, knew people who used it, and knew how to go about getting hold of some for myself. I contacted an anthroposophic doctor in another city, who had treated me once previously, and told her my news. Could she put me in touch with a supplier of *Iscador*?

"Of course," she said, after expressing her sympathy. "We use another brand,

Abdoba. Is that all right with you?" I'm certainly not into the fine distinctions at the point and would probably happily swallow whole berries if she told me to. I tell her that's fine with me. "Come and see me as soon as you feel ready after surgery."

I have explained that I do know a doctor here, who practises homeopathy and is familiar with the anthroposophical approach. He is prepared to take me on, with guidance from someone experienced in this therapy.

"Good. You need someone close at hand."

Yes, I do have what I need. A resource, in her, to draw from later, and a very important one here on my doorstep now.

"All courage to you," she adds, her voice resounding with warmth and vigor over the distances, "and all light!"

I do feel lightened and encouraged after our brief exchange. Strange how a few words can engender strength. I call my local doctor next. He answers the phone himself, and fixes an appointment for the following day. That's something else to be grateful for. I don't have to tackle an official system that often takes several weeks to infiltrate.

As luck, or synchronicity, would have it, I had met Dr. Leonard Owsiany two months previously. He had just moved to the area, a couple of miles from us, and had treated Adam successfully for a nasty bout of post-anaesthesia vomiting. Our children attended the same Waldorf School. We had been planning to get to know one another, since he is a doctor and I am a counselor; both sharing an interest in anthroposophical therapy that might lead to some kind of colleagueship. My cancer simply speeded up our relationship. One of its first positive side-effects.

Lenny is a 20th century Thor, with red-gold hair and enormous vitality, who was then doing a 100-hour a week internship in a local hospital, building a private practice, plus maintaining with his Scots wife, Dorothea, (herself a working nurse and masseure,) five children under the age of nine, an immense collie dog, a pretty large cat, and a wall-cage full of brightly colored birds. He is also an accomplished jazz musician and, to quote him, a "compulsive healer".

"Not too compulsive, I hope," I say, knowing full well where that can lead us, but still extremely grateful he is about to focus his energy and insight on me. I tell him some *Viscum Album* is on its way, but I'll have to learn to inject myself. That won't be easy! I usually faint at the sight of a needle in someone else's hand.

"Dorothea will teach you," he says, and pops to the door to call her in. Threading her way between children and animals, she says she'll inject me herself for as long as it takes me to learn. We live close enough. I suggest I might come after the children leave for school.

"Sounds good to me," says Dorothea – a phrase I am to hear so often from her, imbuing even the most complex situations with an aura of positivity and calm. She withdraws, leaving Lenny and me facing each other across his study brimful of pictures, bottles and books.

"Let's begin, if we may, by your telling me a little of your biography. Ten minutes or so. And could you focus on particular moments of stress or loss that you are aware of."

So, off I go. Stresses and losses abound. I pinpoint the major ones in about seven minutes and sit back, fairly proud of this accomplishment. Lenny is looking pretty grave.

"Have you had *any* joy in your life?" he asks. I chuckle. Told from the dark side, this selective chronicle of the past forty years must appear extremely doom-laden. I hardly recognize it myself.

"Oh yes. My life has been full of joy. . ." In fact, taken as a whole, that is how I remember it. Lenny accepts this, while pointing out that my physical and psychological patterns have, indeed, offered an excellent breeding ground for this disease. I'm not sure I want to know about these patterns right now, especially the undoubtably shady psychological ones. So I comment "Oh really," somewhat airily, and let Lenny continue with whatever he has next in mind.

"Well," he says, "Let's start with a constitutional remedy. *Ignatius*, I think. That will take you back to those stress-points where your life flow got blocked. And *Colcy*s – that's bitter cucumber – for the general fibrocystic tendency."

He suggests I lie down while he administers these.

"You may feel rather labile," he warns me. I ask him what that means and he says: "Well – up and down."

I know homeopathic remedies can have an immediate effect. "You may feel worse before you feel better," physicians often warn. My experience with anthroposophic medicine has been subtler – a general increase, over time, in psycho-spiritual strength as well as physical well being. Now I lie, with several small white pellets under my tongue, wondering if I'll instantly levitate or plunge into suicidal despair. Nothing happens. Lenny reads me a piece on the anthroposophic diet for cancer, which he says is of vital importance now. I listen dreamily to his bedside story, much of which floats past me as dreams so often do.

"Don't worry," he says. "We'll go through this again. It will only depress you, going into hospital." Too right. Imagine asking for any of the foods on this list! I continue vaguely to absorb descriptions of grains, minimal protein, organic vegetables, sun-ripened fruits, honey and certain fats and oils.

"These are to warm you," explains Lenny – for many cancer diets rigorously exclude fats. The great "No-No's" I learn, are vegetables of the nightshade family, (potatoes, tomatoes, peppers, eggplant) and mushrooms which flourish, as does cancer, on somewhat unseemly soil.

"Don't worry," he says again. "The main thing is to enjoy your food. Your life too. Fanaticism is dangerous. Besides," he adds, with a twinkle, "I don't think this is going to kill you." No, lying here cozily, with him in charge, I don't think so either.

He also gives me Silica: "to bring light into the organism", and movingly describes how the inner organs need to converse with each other, but can't see to do so at this point of breakdown in community relations. Silica will light their path again. Well, this may sound pretty fey, but it is an evocative image for me, and generates a tender concern for those poor benighted organs – liver, kidneys, spleen – who have struggled so valiantly to sustain me against the heavy odds I have placed on them through so many years of abuse and neglect.

Finally he makes up a "care package" for me to take to hospital: pills to counter the effect of anaesthesia, a jar of honey-colored ointment to smear on the wound, a large bottle of sloeberry elixir to speed recovery. Dorothea, joining us, tells me to hide these. Have I got a small bag I can zip tightly? I'll be in trouble if any hospital authority discovers them. Sounds like a heretic hiding from the Inquisition. And I suppose those of us who espouse alternatives are heretics these days. Dorothea also asks if I have someone to drive me to the hospital, for she will do so herself if I haven't. With five children? I'm glad to be able to tell her that Cynthia has already offered, and Lulu will be there afterwards.

Leaving the Owsianys, I feel they have woven a safety net of their caring and expertise around me, and that their light, warmth and conversation contain and carry me while we jointly attempt to restore these qualities to my interior world. That's healing, I think to myself, as I drive the short stretch home.

Coming in, I find a letter from a friend, telling me he has to withdraw from a workshop I'm running because he is allergic to my cat and has been seriously ill for the past week. I rage up and down my back yard. After a hefty bout of fury, I make several determined phone calls and, within an hour, have found a new home for the cat – something I should have done several years ago. I sit back, feeling exhausted and complacent. Recalling the dimensions of my wrath, I wonder whether this was "labile" behavior, or merely an appropriate reaction? Whatever: I've clearly been able to take action on a matter I'd left hanging far too long. Cancer, or *Ignatius* – something is beginning to help me sort out priorities.

A few other inner sortings now take place. I discover the world will still keep turning even if I take a few days off! Cynthia is already busy arranging for bushels of spinach and carrots to be brought from a biodynamic farm in Ontario. She will have these washed and stored by my return. Four people call to offer to have Adam to stay. What's left for me to worry about? I'd better find something! Well, there's Adam himself. How is he going to feel when I tell him I have to go to hospital? When I tell him I have cancer? He's bound to be pretty anxious and upset.

"Your operation won't be as bad as mine," he declares proudly.

"No, probably not."

"So why will you need to stay in hospital so long?"

"I guess it's because I'm older, and it's a different operation, of course."

"It may be different. I don't expect it will hurt as much."

"No, probably not. But we'll have to get someone to take care of you."

"I'll be OK. I can go to a friend. Or Cynthia can come here." Grasping the nettle, I add that I have a disease called cancer. Has he ever heard of it?
"Sure. But I don't know what it is."

I tell him it happens when cells in our bodies go wonky, they start behaving differently and, if left to themselves, can be dangerous. I'm having the wonky ones removed. Then I'm going to do a lot of things to make sure I don't get any more. He seems satisfied with this explanation. None of the people we know are likely to look aghast if he tells them about me, but you never know. "Cancer" is still a trigger word.

"I'm going to be fine," I tell him.

"Who said you wouldn't?" He responds tartly. He returns to the theme of the operation itself, which interests him far more.

"Will you be allowed to run? Remember I couldn't run for six weeks!"

"I guess I can run. No-one's told me not to yet."

"See then. My surgery must have been worse than yours will be."

"Mind you," I say, being cast in somewhat the same mold as my son, "I won't be able to use my arm as much."

"Well, you don't like playing basketball anyway. So what's the big deal?"

I know my son. I know his different ways of meeting what he fears. This is not one of them. It may be ignorance or wisdom on his part. And I know he may have fear at other times. After an initial jolt, which is no more than my changing tracks, recognizing I need not carry his burden too, I feel a sudden lightening of heart. No – the biggest deal seems now to be my moral commitment to rake up every single leaf in my backyard in the next three days!

Chapter 5

HOSPITAL

"Hospice, Hospital, hostel, spital, hostage, hostile .... from Latin: Hostia, hostis. A place of refuge; food, with shelter; stranger, an enemy, hence "hostile"; expiatory victim offered to the gods."
— Origins, Eric Partridge.

The night before surgery, I have a dream. *"Jeanie, Adam and I are swimming in a great body of water. It is smooth as silk and an opal-colored haze fills the air. We plunge, dive, float upon and beneath the surface like fish, as if this was our true element. Lissom, weightless, I flip, roll, or lie, miraculously suspended a few feet below the water, gazing through silvery realms, deliciously abandoned, filled with a feeling of wondering delight."* I wake confident of the surgery and moved that Jeanie, (an English friend who had a mastectomy a year ago,) should join me at this time. "And all shall be well," I think, recalling the words of Dame Julian of Norwich on a card from another English friend, "and all manner of things shall be well."

Indeed they are. The surgery itself is a piece of cake; literally and figuratively. A neat slice of flesh is removed, the sides pulled, then stitched together again. Preceding this, however, is admitting myself to hospital at an hour when no sane person is out and about with less than a couple of cups of coffee inside him or her, and enduring procedures that, in any other business would guarantee an immediate loss of customers. (Dame Julian was clearly not referring to life's mundane details in her sense of the ultimate triumph of the benign!)

Perhaps the real reason for not allowing patients to eat or drink after midnight preceding surgery has nothing to do with anaesthesia, but is designed to diminish consciousness and rob us of our fighting power. One cannot rant and rave with a dry mouth, nor storm the corridors with knees that buckle at every step.

I was actually extremely fortunate. Cynthia, (complete with knitting,) had driven me downtown and we sat in a waiting room for an hour or so, while half a dozen people arrived from all over Michigan — most of them elderly — to discover their surgery had been cancelled, but no-one had bothered to let them know! They were treated to free breakfasts before they drove a hundred or so miles home again, but it's a long way to drive for breakfast, particularly of the type and quality a hospital provides.

I instantly set about discovering if my own surgery had been cancelled and found it had not, but would be running late. I'd figured this out for myself, for by this time I should have been lying somewhere attached to an IV, instead of wistfully hoping someone might notice me. Several people do notice me, actually. They variously test my heart, record my next of kin, rent me a TV – but none are remotely concerned with the operation itself and eventually I suggest to the receptionist that I find my way to the pre-operating room. (What a difference it would make if patients were shown their rooms, knew there was a space waiting for them to come home to. But this is not to be.) Cynthia and I lug my bags, and her knitting, down several flights of stairs to a narrow room reminiscent of the London Underground in wartime, piled deep with people, standing room only at this point. We continue to wait until I notice I am the only person wearing an identification tab and call the attention of a passing nurse to enquire if I should be somewhere else.

"Sure," she says. "Just get undressed and come through this door when you're ready." So I scuffle out of my clothes as modestly as I can behind a curtain and put on a robe that covers about a quarter of me, so all modesty is pretty pointless, as I scuttle past all the people again, (still with my baggage,) and finally enter the arena I've been aiming for; suitably sterile, filled with metal and plastic contraptions and green-robed figures discussing their dates or the latest basketball scores.

The waiting continues, this time horizontally, which is about all I am fit for by now. No-one tells me why we are delayed. There's ample time to imagine setbacks in the preceding patient – some ghastly, uncalculated turn of events. I decide it is better not to imagine, but to lie mindlessly, one of a sacrificial row of victims, robed in white, but still with too few blankets and frozen feet. (What would it cost a hospital to issue warm woolly stockings, even a hot water bottle, to ease these long hours? Is this a "place of refuge"? Or are we indeed the "expiatory victims offered to the gods"? And, if so, to which gods, and for what sins?)

In between meditating on such questions, I receive a few visitors, who plug things in, take X-rays, and so forth. There's a perilous moment when I foolishly let slip to an intern who has paused to practise his bedside manner, that I am taking Silica. He snaps out his notebook to record this and I imagine the surgery suspended, and hospital administrators descending like storm troopers to evict me from the premises.

"You can take it as a herbal tea," I tell the intern wildly.

"*Equisitum* – horsetail. Just horsetail. Maybe you've heard of it?" He hasn't. I decline to add that I read recently of a dog that developed cancer on too high a dosage – so much for meek and mild homeopathy. But if people, (by whom I mean conventional medicos,) don't believe it does us any good, I'm certainly not going to let on that it can do harm, if wrongly prescribed, and is as potent as many of the chemicals they administer! The rest of my natural pharmocopoeia is tidily tucked in my overstay bag. I'll take it, like a secret addict, in whatever private moments I can snatch in the following days. Mercifully, he snaps his notebook shut again.

Well, this too passes, and within a few hours, most of which go unrecorded by me while Pamela does her work, I am tucked up in the neurological ward: "No room for you where you're meant to be", and have kicked up enough fuss to discover where Lulu is and got her from there to beside me. No nice cup of tea, or even a glass of water. But on the dot of 6 o'clock, supper arrives.

I'm pretty sure hospitals, like prisons, have an overcrowding problem and solve it quite simply by producing food (so-called) that either drives you home as soon as you can stagger up, or kills you off. It's probably a collusion between them and medical insurance companies. Or it may be that hospitals know their name shares a root origin with the word "hostile" and feel pledged to honor this. Whichever fantasy we choose, the food is unfailingly revolting. I am sure my hospital is no better or worse than others the world over, and bemused patients in Baghdad or Bolivia are served a similar fare: to wit: meat in three shapes (cube, circle and rectangle, with frilly sections of fat glued on where appropriate) and in two colors – beige or brown: vegetables that clearly never saw earth and have spent at least forty hours in tepid dishwater: and truly gory desserts such as puce or viridian jello. This awe-inspiring offering now confronted me when I lifted the plastic covers on my plastic tray and unleashed smells I would rather not dwell on here. Lulu and I take one look, and I break my first pre-surgical resolution within an hour of returning consciousness.
"Let's go to the lounge and have coffee and a cigarette."
So off we go, trundling a large metal contraption attached to my IV, and Lulu fetches coffee from the visitors' cafeteria because we don't trust the stuff for patients, and we sit looking out at the sun setting over the city and celebrate the passing of this first trial.

There are further trials to come. That night I find myself sharing a room with Bessie, an elderly black woman who is tied to her bed with tubes in every orifice. When conscious, she is in a state of deep terror. She implores me to sever her bonds. "I know you have a knife, darling. I can see its shadow on the wall." Much though I would like to set her free, I daren't risk it for her sake.
"Oh Lord, oh Lord," she moans, "Oh Lord, save me." In the darkness, I heave myself out of bed and lug my metal companion with me to the foot of hers.
"Hey, Bessie. I'm here."
"Oh, Lord," she whimpers, her eyes closed, her arms scrabbling in the empty air beyond her bonds. I can't even reach her hand, with all the paraphanalia that surrounds us, so I sit on the edge of her bed, murmuring helplessly:
"Hey, Bessie, take it easy now."
But she continues to call on the Lord as indeed I am inwardly doing too, and her voice rises and falls in something like the beginning of song. Listening a few moments, I ask:
"Can you sing to the Lord, Bessie? Can you sing to Him?"
Yes, she can. From some deep region her voice swells in an urgent gospel

of suffering and appeal. I listen to her rough, anguished, lovely voice till it sinks to a murmur, her breathing steadies, and at last she drops off into a blessed sleep. And so, indeed, do I.

It is at this point that Staff Nurse arrives. She wears tap dancing shoes. Talk about "presence"; you can sense her half a mile away – bustle, bustle thump, squeak. "Well, Bessie," she cries loudly, entering the room and flinging curtains and trays out of her way.

"And how are *we* doing?" Bessie was fine, with the Lord Jesus, till she came. So what is nurse's problem?

"Hi, Bessie!" she cries again, standing at the foot of the bed.

"Tell us now. Who is President of the United States?"

Bessie groans – an entirely appropriate response in my view.

"Don't remember? Well then, Bessie, what year is it?"

Further wise groans and mutterings. It appears Bessie does not know or care what day or month it is. At 3am, her time is now, eternal, eternally terrible.

"See," says nurse triumphantly, coming to my bed to make sure she's woken me to hear and witness this.

"She's quite out of it. We'll move you tomorrow." Even if I groan at the mention of the President's name? I must remember that's the litmus test here for madness or sanity.

I am indeed moved the following day, and I certainly sleep better, though I am haunted by the thought of Bessie, whom I learn has also been moved and I may never see again. Dori, snatching moments she can ill afford between school, work, family life, brings me brown rice and crunchy vegetables. Paul sends, at my request, five cigarettes, (I am now in a room with a chain smoker;) one for each day and one to spare. I relish these in the patients' lounge, together with some fine and interesting encounters. Patrick, who works at the Belle Isle conservatory, comes shyly in with a rare, extravagant, waxy white bloom. Adam visits on his way home from school. He calls twice, on his own initiative, and hearing his high clear voice over the phone is better than a five-star meal. Lenny and Dorothea are continually in touch, full of interest and encouragement. Lenny offers to visit me, if I need him. But I feel fine, slugging down my elixir furtively in between the bustling, squeaking visits of nurses and orderlies. Many others call. We have rich, funny conversations. Oh, what a company. And how I thank you all.

Pamela Benitez visits me every day. She is unfailingly cheerful, despite what seems to me an appalling schedule, compounded by driving from her home in Ann Arbor through wintry weather. She tells me with as much delight as if it had been her own cancer that my lymph nodes were free of malignancy. She had managed to capture seventeen of them in the fairly small slice she removed, which I gather was no mean feat. Rather like our British Good Friday ritual, when we close our eyes and hope to get a mouthful of currants as we bite into our hot cross buns! Good for her. I wouldn't know a lymph note if one came to call. She seems

pleased with her handiwork too. I squint down cautiously between the gauze wrappings at a web of black stitches and my nipple keeling at a shipwrecked angle in a sea of bruised flesh. I'm not ready for close-ups yet. I don't feel ready for much of anything and, when I say, rather wistfully, that it will be lovely when I can take a bath and wash my hair, I am quite horrified by her reply.
"Any time. Have a shower now if you want."
She'd probably give the OK if I wanted to pilot a transatlantic flight. Though I instantly decide a shower is not imperative, Pamela strongly urges me to visit the ROC (Radiation Oncology Center) while I am here on the premises.

She fixes an appointment and on my third day I am wheeled along corridors to that stately dome in my flannel nightgown and frayed Marks & Spencer's dressing gown. This is truly the Zanadu of the medical complex; an astonishing confection of sugar pink pillars and glass domes, at the heart of four surrounding hospitals, along whose dark, converging tunnels like veins and arteries, patients are perpetually pumped to and fro.

My interview with a particular doctor at the ROC may well have planted the seed of doubt about radiation that was to take root over the following weeks.

She was brisk, competent, thorough. She gave me every fact I sought, and several I did not. She spared time for all my questions, at least for those I was able to formulate, and offered to be available should others occur to me later. She had a large hole in her stocking which endeared her to me. But there were no holes in her presentation. She even took the trouble to assure me that there was no conclusive evidence as yet to suggest that radiating the breast could cause lung cancer! I was, according to her, an optimum case for her treatment: so early was my cancer that this was just the time to swipe it before it knew what had hit it. Recurrence was highly unlikely (98% against), but almost a certainty if I neglected this step, which fitted the surgery I had had like a buckskin glove to the hand.

She was a very compelling saleswoman, describing in loving detail the tailor-made cup that would cover what remained of my breast and allow the rays to angle in at various depths and intensities. She clearly believed in her product, which began to sound like an advertisement for the most delicate and luxurious brassiere. There were clearly no alternatives in her mind. When I suggested some: diet, homeopathy, visualization, these impressed her as little as if I were to suggest to an *haute couturier* that I join a nudist colony, and I soon stopped mentioning them.
"So you think that I'm a high risk if I refuse?"
"Yes, I know you are a high risk."
"And if I leave it a while and come later, say in a year's time?"
"I won't treat you. The situation will have changed too much."
So that's how it was. I was wheeled back again. My bed almost seemed like home. I snuggled down under the thin covers and, yes, actually covered my head.
"But she was quite fair, quite reasonable," I argued with myself – the self that said plainly:
"I don't like that place. It's cold, and I feel cold."

Later, I tackle my resistance, including the bit that invariably balks at the American hard sell. I explore other centers. I become quite knowledgeable about dosages, rads, the equipment used, (learning incidentally, that the latter is highly significant, since antiquated machinery may well zap the cancer, but could leave your breast hard as a rock!) I read the Simonton's book, *Getting Well Again*. Yes, I'm sure I could make a positive relationship with the machine, christen it Arnold, evoke delightful imagery. But do I want to? That remains the question, and I put it on hold, as I generally do the tough, unanswerable ones.

The remaining days pass uneventfully. Dorothea had supplied me with several good novels – a welcome alternative to the exclusive diet of soap operas and sitcoms American TV provides. I begin to master the drain; a tube inserted near my armpit, dripping fluid into a little plastic bag that Pamela assures me I can tuck artfully into my waistband as soon as I feel ready to go home. And soon I do feel ready – quite proud, in fact, that I have the confidence to deal with the drain on my own. Dori fetches me, a one-armed bandit, feeling both nurtured and faintly ridiculous as she carries my bags to the car.

At home, all is quiet. Adam is not due back for another couple of hours. I sit in a pool of golden silence, filled with flowers that have mysteriously arrived and been arranged by some loving hand. I walk the sunny winter streets, breathing cold, delicious air. There's a pile of mail: cards and letters from many friends. I breathe in these messages too, and weep a little for joy. This is true radiation. This, too, is not easy to bear. But I make a space in myself, and their words fill it with another golden light.

How did Lulu find time, between driving me everywhere, to copy the following, that becomes my guiding image, crystallizing this time of return, this time of a new beginning?

"What I am trying to say is hard to tell and hard to understand . . . . unless, unless, you have yourself been at the edge of the Deep Canyon and have come back unharmed. Maybe it all depends on something within yourself – whether you are trying to see the Watersnake or the Sacred Cornflower, whether you go out to meet death or to seek life. It is like this; as long as you walk at the very edge of the Deep Canyon, you may indeed stay within the realm of the great Cloudbeings and not be harmed. You will be protected by the rainbow and the Great Ones. You will have no reason to worry and no reason to be sad. You may fight with witches and if you can meet them with a heart that does not tremble, the fight will make you stronger. It will help you to attain your goal in life. It will give you strength to help others, to be loved and liked, and to seek life."
May you stay within the realm of the great Cloudbeings. Welcome home, Lulu.

Yes, may we all stay within the realm of the Great Cloudbeings, I think, as I fall asleep that night.

Chapter 6

FIRST STEPS

"If one moves forward, one is bound to encounter something!"
— I Ching

Now follow quiet days. Even the earth stills, beginning to hold its breath for winter. The air is sharp and bright. How curious, I reflect, that my life has carved a space for this event. After the rush of the past weeks, it, too, has become empty and still.

Work has fallen away quite naturally. No more clients come. Perhaps intuitively I had barely enrolled in September for my religious studies program at Marygrove. When I call my tutor, Mary-Ellen, to explain this turn of events, she understands completely. This is no time to study religion. Perhaps a time for living more religiously. She takes me into her prayers, and asks if I am willing for my name to be included in a healing Mass. Of course I am. What a strong and lovely branch of my "Tree" she is.

So beyond taking care of Adam, I have nothing to do but heal myself. Or be healed. Or both. It's clear that this is a joint enterprise.

My mother arrives. So does my bottle of *Viscum Album*. I hold the little vial, full of a slightly pearly substance, as if it were a treasure only to be found in fairy tales. The Water of Life? Perhaps it is. I am certainly eager for my first dose of it.

We call Dorothea and my mother drives me to the Owsianys. I'm quite capable of driving myself, but slightly nervous of getting the tubing from my drain wound round the gear shift, and even more nervous that the mistletoe may have some lightning effect on me, as the *Ignatius* did not. Besides, I want my mother to meet Dorothea. I feel knowing my healers will reassure her. In fact, she is highly supportive of my choices so far, and had arrived laden with books full of fascinating accounts of alternative healings by a number of British folk.

Unlike Americans, the British have not lost touch with many natural healing practices. Our Queen is President of the Homeopathic Hospital in London. Herbalism, naturopathy, as well as homeopathy, were somewhat submerged in the waves of "scientific" materialism, but never wholly drowned. It is customary to this day to enquire at a country chemist (drug store) if anyone who can charm warts lives nearby. (In France, you simply ask for the nearest witch!) So neither of us are new to this sort of thing. But the power of the medical model still goes deep. She knows I'm still grappling with the question of radiation, and have been

31

told by one "expert" that without it I'm a lost cause. We also both know that mistletoe offers no miracles. It may not be able to turn around the cancer at this stage. But at least she'll experience how closely supported I am by people. Who else can go prancing off each morning to have an injection, (no charge), surrounded by children and singing birds?

Gideon, the dog, is waiting at the door. Sarah, age four, and Kirstin, age two, take charge of my mother, while Dorothea fetches a syringe and takes me into Lenny's office, quickly locking the door. "Kirsti's in a breaking-and-entering phase," she explains. "Into everything! And she'll probably start shrieking now." All is quiet. "Well, I wonder what happened," says Dorothea. "She always shrieks." "It's my mother," I say. She'll be telling Kirstin her giant stories, that captivate Adam to this day. Dorothea takes my vial and fills the syringe.

"Into the breast first, I think," she says. "We'll work later along the line of surgery. You probably feel pretty tender there now."

I do. But it's a strange thing. I feel so positive about the mistletoe that I'm ready to have it anywhere. Never has an injection been so welcomed. I already imagine its healing powers suffusing me. Dorothea gently injects me – I feel nothing – and tells me to lie still for a while to let it take effect. She leaves to put the kettle on.

After fifteen minutes or so, she returns.

"Well, how are you feeling?"

"Fine. I don't feel anything." Am I a hard nut to crack? I had rather hoped for a splendid reaction, and feel a flicker of disappointment that nothing seems to have changed.

"It may take a while," says Dorothea, comfortingly. "And it's a low dose. It affects everyone differently."

The most common symptoms are increased temperature, perhaps feeling flu-like, and some redness or swelling at the injection site. Perhaps my soul was so receptive to the mistletoe that my body has received it with equal happiness? I must now begin to monitor my temperature regularly twice a day, particularly noticing if it rises within a few hours of the injection. Dorothea suggests I lie down again when I get home. These resting periods are a distinctive feature of my therapies, as I am to learn as I go along. The body is given no distractions, to allow the effect of its encounter with the remedy or therapy to work more deeply. During these times I am encouraged to think of nothing, to let my mind go blank, so that my consciousness does not divert and erode forces that have other work to do. This is hard. I'm not used to lying inert, with an emptied mind. I'd rather scrub a floor or make a shopping list. I'd even rather meditate! So I learn, simply through these passive moments, some deep truths about my own pathology, as the tendencies that have in part led to this illness are mirrored back to me.

*   *   *

I am aware that the question of radiation still hovers over me. I cannot empty my mind of that. I talk with Dorothea, whose own mother had radiation many years ago. She is definitely not against it herself. The following mornings, she brings out heavy medical textbooks, full of statistics and photographs. I notice how often I forget to bring my glasses, so I can't read a word of the small print. Nor can I see, beyond a general blur, the gruesome pictures of advanced breast cancer, where cauliflower growths have broken through the skin. I ask Lenny, too, who is sometimes home after a night shift at the hospital. He also thinks it might be a good idea.

"We don't want to run any risks," he says. "It's an effective treatment, and we can always lessen the side effects with homeopathy."

This depresses me. Is he saying he has no faith in the mistletoe, or indeed his own pharmocopoeia? And why is it that others now call to ask me – albeit lovingly – not to reject it out of hand? Nancy, whose intuitions I trust so deeply: Jane, whose own son's life was prolonged so many years because of it. Are these messages I am meant to hear as my answer, or is the challenge for me to stand against them with conviction?

I return to my image of healing – "to make whole". Conventional treatments scarcely do that. They actually honor the belief that it is the body that heals itself, also of the destruction wrought upon it by them. Of course destruction has its place. All creation moves between the poles of life and death. Our bodies continually break down substances to generate new energies. We prune trees, weed gardens, to encourage appropriate growth. It seems a matter of when, and what and how much any living organism can bear. I considered the nature of the particular treatments for cancer, striving to get some sense of what I could take on, what I personally might bear.

Surgery is the most visibly destructive, excising tumors, often removing large areas of healthy tissue surrounding them. As Bernie Siegel points out in *Love, Medicine & Miracles*, this is not a cure. It simply buys us time, removing the immediate threat to our health while we consider ways of restoring and maintaining it – rather like ousting a robber at gunpoint, before we look to what may protect house and home if we live in a high risk area. Once cancer has manifest, we are certainly at high risk. I was grateful for my own surgery; the time it might have bought me. And, knowing how slow I am to make changes, perhaps I needed the further protection radiation might give?

Radiation appears to consolidate the work of surgery. Both cancerous and benign cells are destroyed over a specific area in the hope that only benign ones will replace them. In my case, with pretty advanced fibrocystic breast disease, there was a high probability that additional cells were lurking here and there. And I understood that the surgery itself juggled things up, so the robbers could all too easily make their escape to other premises.

Why wouldn't I choose this treatment? I had been assured that I would feel nothing at all. The only effect might be something resembling sunburn. I might feel tired, but far less so than if I had chemotherapy which is, to put it bluntly, a systemic poisoning. In this, the drugs zap all the quickest growing and multiplying cells throughout the body, taking billions of healthy ones. Thus hair falls out, moist body areas dry up – not to mention how sick and exhausted most patients feel while on this treatment. Some of the enduring side-effects people had told me about were actually attributable to the treatment, not the disease itself.

A mere fifteen minutes lying under a machine daily for five weeks, with virtually no pain or discomfort, seems a very low price to pay for additional insurance against the spread of my disease.

Yet, still I balked. And, paradoxically, it was often the sense that this treatment was so invisible, intangible, that most disturbed me. I was haunted by an exchange I had with the doctor at the ROC when I asked her in passing if she thought the numbed area surrounding my surgery would ever regain feeling, since I imagined difficulties shaving under my arm.
"Oh," she replied happily, "You probably won't ever grow hair there after radiation." For her this was clearly a super bonus; for me, a deeply shocking awareness of the true nature of this treatment. I realized I was very afraid of those lethal, invisible rays. Though I don't like meeting nasty things, I'd always prefer to meet them face to face!

My mother and I discussed the issue frequently. I'd been given one set of statistics and they sounded impressive. I argued, however, that the five-year "promise" of health most likely reflected the earlier diagnosis of cancer: in other words, it normally took five years or so to spread. I suggested that such statistics embody the half-truth that may be worse than a lie, encouraging the illusory belief that we can, within some margin of error, predict our fate. One of the gifts of a life-threatening illness is that it faces us fair and square with the truth that we cannot know, from one hour to the next, what may befall us. I chuckled, imagining choosing radiation as a sure-fire cure and meeting my end driving to a session on the icy roads of midwinter Michigan. No, statistics clearly failed to impel me either way!

So, we, and others, batted the question back and forth. Each time I felt it would be a wise choice, another factor would sway the balance. The day my mother and I ran through a scenario that delightfully included my friend Judith flying from England to support me through those five weeks, Pamela Benitez called to tell me she had just attended a conference in which a group of oncologists and radiologists couldn't decide if radiation had any value at all! I did honestly wish at times I was either a Christian Scientist, or believed that everything outside the medical establishment was witchcraft and quackery. I did wish, too, that there were not so many levels to the question. It was not merely a matter of survival for the next few decades, but contained deeper issues of long-term consequences. Was my motive to prolong my life at any cost? Why should I imagine I owed it to Adam – not to mention myself or the world? Might Adam's own destiny unfold more fruitfully without me? All these reflections were endless and, of course, unanswerable. All I could come to was that I would not hurry this choice. There was surely some radiation therapist in the northern hemisphere who would treat me if I let a month or so elapse?

As an interim alternative, I throw my first Radiation Party. I'm not certain my mother, or indeed a few friends, think this is in very good taste! Am I joking about matters that should be taken more seriously? Actually, I do feel quite serious. An exchange of healing rays between us may be far more potent than those emitted by those glittering, cold machines.

We prepare lots of tasty munchies that substantially exclude the "No-No's" of my diet, and make a blazing fire. The room is still full of wonderful flowers. We light lots of candles too. In out of the cold night air they come: Karen and Paul, Cynthia and John, Mary-Jo, Rob, Cammie, Reg. Others follow behind. We gather round the fire, eat, drink, talk, above all, laugh! At previous parties I've raced around, fueled by coffee and cigarettes, feeling it's up to me to get fresh drinks and hand out plates or the whole precarious edifice might well collapse. Tonight, I curl up on the sofa, nursing my drain, in a delightful, receptive euphoria. The lack of stimulants has something to do with it. Unfocused, I silently absorb the presence of this warming, light-filled company. Stronger than Silica perhaps?

After they leave, I sleep such a grace-filled sleep in which these friends flow through my dreams, the echo of their laughter reverberating in me. Yes, I feel truly radiated. I hope they all do too. What happens to one of us surely touches us all?

Chapter 7

VOICES

"For the word to be spoken, there must be silence – before and after."
— The Farthest Shore, Ursula Le Guin.

Marjanna had written: "Listen to your angel. He is very close at these times." Marjanna, who had breast cancer a year ago, is ahead of me on this journey and can send reports on weather and terrain to one who has just set forth. Though I spend quiet times, in meditation or prayer, I am only subliminally aware of her injunction, and no voice sounds in these spaces – at least that I can hear. I may feel peace, a rush of courage; messages indeed from an unseen world; yet no clear pronouncement is forthcoming, and any I think I hear sound a great deal like my own voice – all too familiar, saying the kinds of things I want or need to hear.

But one day, busy in the kitchen cutting carrots, I am knocked sideways by the words: "You can live twenty years." I almost look round, expecting a physically incarnate visitor. I mutter, feeling very foolish: "What did you say?" The voice, like an echo, repeats itself. I sit down abruptly. Did I really hear that or not? I ask again. All is silent. That, as much as anything, authenticates the occurrence, though what or who spoke is still questionable. Some might call it the voice of the Self, (which Carl Jung also called the God within.) Some might call it God. I thought it might be my guardian angel. God surely delegates much to other beings in His service. For lack of evidence to the contrary, I stick with that.

I stand by, thereafter, for further messages, rather like tuning in a ham radio in some beleaguered country, but all I get is silence or crackling wires. At times I feel demanding and cheated. "Here am I, all set, plugged in. What's keeping you?" Finally, I let go of need or desire.

When my mother arrives, her presence amply compensates for the lack of discarnate beings. Her voice and being has sustained me through many years. I drop the other business and settle in to some good conversations with her instead.

After the radiation party, and a stupendous Thanksgiving feast with friends, we plan a trip to Point Pelée in southern Ontario, with Adam and Mary-Jo, to introduce my mother to another side of living in the grim, so often desperate city of Detroit. Point Pelée is one of our "power" places that several of us visit as often as we have the opportunity.

36

Here a tapering triangle of land juts into Lake Erie like the last or first firmament, set upon waters that pulse and break against it; sometimes changing its contours, yet never reclaiming it. Emerging from woodlands filled with rare plants and creatures, on to this low naked spit of sand, I have often gasped to see its tip submerged by ice or white waves – yet, in another season, it always returns. Here birds rest on their long migrations, and the Monarch butterflies pause in thousands on their long journey from north and east to New Mexico. This place offers a pause for refreshment for all who come here in mid-flight. It seems that the membrane between visible and invisible worlds thins to transparency; that what manifests as rock or shell, cloud, wave, or vertical shaft of light, are merely intense concentrations of invisible force and energy. Contemplating these, one may slip effortlessly across a threshold into other dimensions of reality.

On this bright still silent November day we walk through bare thickets towards the lake like a silver mirror; so calm, so glassy, it holds on its wide surface all the patterns of light and air above. Its silence silences us. Its stillness stops us in our tracks. As I bend to touch a stone, I hear the voice again. This time it says: "Love the earth." I cock my ear and hear the echo, faint yet unmistakable as ocean sounding in a shell. When I try to summon it once more, only my words come. A great and terrible tenderness breaks over me. Each pebble, each shell, is filled with beauty; each, in this moment, articulate, a word spoken, and I imagine beyond the grasp of hearing the great murmuring of creation beneath my feet. I feel these patient stones lie like an eternal sacrifice, offering me the ground of their existence on which to grind and crunch the pathways of my life. Thus have I done – regardless, indifferent – for over forty years!

Thinking this I turn to bush and tree. Stripped to the bone now, they offer the shapes of their skeletons to my awareness; each joint and limb distinct, unique. Have I ever truly noticed them before? Now surely, one step closer, one glance deeper, and I'll see the world that weaves within them and about them. And it seems important that I do. Imperative that I see, touch, taste, smell, through all their cycles of growth and death. It feels they call me into connection, not only with their visible presence – bud, leaf, blossom, seed, – but also with the spirits who wear these as a garment, who wait with infinite patience for my knowing them. I have not begun. I haven't begun to love the earth. Does it take the awareness of our death to wake us up to life?

When we come home, a wave of anguish builds in me and I sob in my mother's arms. "I want to do the *moral* thing." Do either of us know what I mean? It feels important to speak these words; far more important than cancer, far more important than whether I live or die. And it is to my mother that I need to speak. Not merely because she is the one who is there. Nor yet because she has been, since before I can remember, the comforter towards whom I, the child, turned. No, she is the particular spirit who may hear, behind the words spoken, what I am trying to tell, where I am trying to go.

The voice has one more word to say. It says; "Listen". It says "listen" as I walk the snowy streets, heave bags and baskets from the grocery store. When I babble to friends, the word "listen" is thrown like a rock in a running stream. It whispers "listen" while I bend over the face of my sleeping child. And when I go out a last time to see stars burning in the winter night, "listen" sounds down from each of them, reverberating across the immeasurable distances to beat tenderly, yet insistently, upon my wondering heart. "Listen" and "Love the Earth". Simple, yet great commands. I had better live twenty years if I am to begin to learn how to obey them!

Chapter 8

DOCTORS

"My child, when you are ill, do not rebel,
but pray to the Lord, and he will heal you.
Then let the doctor take over –
The Lord created him too."

— Ecclesiastes 38:1,9

Lenny and Dorothea remove my drain. Pamela had told me I could do this myself. Her confidence in me is delightful, but in this instance somewhat misplaced. I discover one evening that my left side is soaking wet. The drain has overflowed. I panic, and call the Owsianys, who tell me to come right over, no problem, this happens frequently. Well, I get enough blocked household drains, so why not this one? Tucking me up on their couch, they tell me to hold my breath and, with a pop and a slither, out it comes in Lenny's capable hands. "What a sucker!" he exclaims. "Just take a look at that." I turn my head cautiously. The end that was inserted under my skin is the size of a large cigarette holder pressed flat. Thank God I didn't know that before!

"Well, now you're ready to travel," says Lenny. "You'll probably have a bigger scar from this than from the quandrantectomy." He admires Pamela's handiwork. Also *Symphytum*, the golden ointment I have been smearing over the wound, has speeded the healing process remarkably. Lenny tells me a surgeon had called him recently to express wonder at another patient's recovery from surgery due to this and other homeopathic treatment.

"You may get a fluid build-up," cautions Dorothea. "But not to worry. That's quite normal, and can easily be drained off." "Not to worry," is another of Dorothea's expressions that goes hand in hand with "sounds good to me". Her calmness is as infectious as Lenny's vigor. What a good match and complement they are to each other. And I can draw from both.

So I am ready to travel. To Chicago to visit the anthroposophic doctor there. I remember her as a small, strong, quick woman, with warmth and humor, sharing her practice with her husband above a drug store and thrift shop in a comfortably shabby neighborhood. Irene comes with me, bless her. She wants a consultation too, and actually looks more depleted than I.

It is quite a journey by bus and the El, through a heavy downpour, and we need to recuperate in the thrift shop. There's nothing that elevates the spirit so quickly

39

as a few good bargains. I hope the doctor doesn't prescribe too many medicines, for I won't be able to carry them as well as the boots, shirts and pants I stagger out with after this successful spree.

"Well, you look as though you've been through something," she says, appraising me shrewdly, when we are together in her light and spacious consulting room. I don't know whether to feel upset or pleased. I thought I looked rather splendid – though damp – with a new golden glow under my skin, induced by a daily gallon or so of carrot juice. But it is nice to know someone sees below the surface, for I have been through something, and still have a long way through to go.

"So," she continues, when we are seated comfortably. "God's given you a tap on the shoulder, has He, to turn your life around?"

"A bloody great thump, if you ask me!"

"Well, you haven't lost your humor. Good. You'll need that." She asks me about the surgery, and glances through my pathology reports and copies of my mammogram.

"Let's take a look at you – if you don't mind." I don't. I'm always struck by the tact such a doctor shows towards physical examination, that so subtly dignifies the event for me. Also, I am amazed by what she finds, sees, through her fingertips. Last visit she told me it felt as though I'd had three incarnations rolled into one; and that deduced by gently probing the soles of my feet!

Now she moves her hand quietly, delicately, over my breast, my scar, and a tennis-ball lump under my arm.

"Is that a tumor?" She asks.

"No!" I squawk, terror welling up in my stomach. "I mean, it's fluid, isn't it? It's only fluid. Isn't that all it is?"

"I don't know," she says. "Ask your surgeon. Question, question, question! Ask about everything!" Oh, my God. Whatever precarious sense of confidence I felt till now begins to slip. I clutch the edge of the examining table and, on the verge of tears, say self-piteously: "I want nine years. Till my son is grown. At least nine years."

"You may have many more than that," she responds tartly. "You'll probably still be around at eighty, so you'd better be prepared for it!"

She increases my dosage of Silica: "Light. Light, we need." And gives me a potent strain of Acidophilus. When I tell her I have a milder one at home, she briskly rejects it.

"We don't play Mickey Mouse with this thing." She tells me how to monitor the effect of the mistletoe more closely, draw up temperature charts, and sets me up for an abstruse blood test which only a laboratory in Orange County, California will do. I will have to Federal Express four vials of blood, so they can do a full breakdown on lymphocytes, killer cells, as well as a host of other things.

I ask what she thinks about radiation. She looks at me strangely, and hesitates before replying.

"I don't know that you should be asking me," she says finally. "I must admit I have a strong personal prejudice."

She explains that while working in a cancer clinic, with many dying patients, she was struck by something difficult about the deaths of those who had had radiation in the past.

"They seemed to die too fast," she said, yet I could feel her remembering and struggling for some objectivity. She adds firmly: "This was only my experience. Others might see it very differently."

She clearly means to leave me free, which simply means more confused! If one has to die, wouldn't it be good to do so as fast as possible? Why won't some voice boom down from heaven telling me what to do?

She concludes our interview with a further complexity, suggesting that if I am to continue treatment through this practice it might be better if her husband took me on. He is – as I well know – a great authority on cancer and this therapy. "I don't want to turn you out," she adds, "but it might be better this way." But I do feel rejected, and embarrassingly close to tears again at the prospect of being abandoned to some stranger, however expert he may be.

Staggering back to the airport in rush hour, through the unending rain, miserably aware I haven't eaten properly all day, I feel crushed by our encounter. Shouldn't she have gone a little lighter on me? Given me a hug, or something? She was supposed to make me feel better, not worse! Yet, later, I wonder if her toughness wasn't deliberate. She may have been testing my courage and will. For, within days, my fighting spirit has returned. My blood is up. I question, challenge, demand. Pamela examines my tennis ball and pronounces it to be fluid. It begins to dissolve. I barge about, insisting on copies of lab reports, speaking to radiation centers, tackling medical text books – and, through all this, wondering, rather furiously, what or where I am supposed to turn my life towards. I inform God that he'd better buck up and tell me, because I certainly don't know! Yet, even questing through all my available resources, I still feel in the little league as a cancer expert, and when Pamela suggests I talk to an oncologist, I agree this is probably the next step.

"She's a strong woman," says Pamela – no slouch herself.

"I think you'll get along together pretty well." Dr. Silvana Martino is her name. This inspires hope in me, even before we meet. Were her name not enough, she is also credited with being one of the top oncologists in this city, and I hear her praises from others while waiting for my first interview.

Same hospital. Same purple, lime-green and orange chairs in the waiting room. Same bleak procedures: unrobing, being weighed, waiting like a plate of chilled cold cuts in a stark, angular cubicle. But when Dr. Martino enters, the resemblance ends. Her voice is full of music, her eyes warm, brown, direct. She brings a sense of time and space with her that surrounds us both, and makes of that harsh white box an intimate meeting place.

"What a beautiful name you have," I tell her. "Are you from Italy?"
"We came from a little mountain village there," she says.   I begin to smile,
remembering my own time spent there; the smells, textures, colors of that land;
olive and cypress, baked earth, dark wine drunk in some village cafe with a view
that, in places, is unchanged since Piero della Francesca painted it. Let's go there
now, and forget medical matters. Italy is probably a cure for cancer anyhow!
      But we continue here.   Dr. Martino explores my breast and body with a
questing, reverent touch. She is sensing with more than her hands, I know. I feel
imagination working here – of the true kind. I hear it in the pictures she brings of
this disease, answering all my questions with images. Now I can relax, as a child
might, listening to a story that touches not just mind, but heart. I do feel like a child
here, in the best possible way, as she tells me she thinks of cancer cells as aliens –
one can destroy them, return them to their own country, or maybe even incorporate
them into the community if they can learn its laws, its modes of behavior.
"So what have you decided to do?"
      I tell her about the mistletoe – which interests her, and my reluctance to zap
my body with radiation; my preference for what I would call immune-therapy.
"I thought you might say that," she says, with a twinkle in those nice brown eyes.
"But sometimes I worry that I'm not afraid enough," I confess. "Maybe I'm being
very stupid?"
"Maybe you know there's nothing to fear," she replies. She takes a deep breath,
and says tentatively:
"I hope you don't mind my saying this.   Some people don't like religious
terminology. But I sometimes feel God touches us through an illness. He brings
us an illness as an opportunity to grow, to change."
      Whoa there, Lady! Aren't I the one supposed to be saying that? Aren't you
the scientific materialist; quantifying, analyzing specks of matter, and brewing up
another bunch of specks to administer intravenously? I smile again. I begin to
breathe more deeply than I've ever breathed in this building before. "Don't talk
to the establishment," I recall someone saying, "they don't understand. They'll
reject you, and it will only make things worse." But here, in this woman, streams
can meet: science and art; the conventional and the alternative. Here we, as
people, can meet. It is people, of course, far more than medicines, that really heal.
She's one of them.
      So I can mention that I need to look, too, for what is cancerous in my soul;
what is split-off, living its life apart, at the expense of the totality. Yes, she agrees.
"So does anyone offer that sort of thing here, at this clinic, to your customers?"
"No, not much yet. If you ever get anything started, let me know." She adds that
she would like to see any studies I can obtain on the mistletoe treatment, and
expresses interest in the particular features of the diet I'm on. Then I dare ask the
question that has really been hovering over me for the past twenty minutes or so.
"If I refuse radiation, will you still see me?"
"Yes."

"Oh. I was told doctors wouldn't, if I didn't follow what's recommended."
"But I will."

After our session, she takes me to meet Cyndi, her assistant. I am introduced as the Mistletoe Lady. I drive home on the freeway, singing. Yes, it is people who heal – or the encounter between people; what happens in between. Maybe we won't beat the cancer, but is it for this alone that I seek a cure?

* * *

There is one more journey to make before my therapeutic team is complete. Lenny suggests I visit an anthroposophic doctor in Pennsylvania, whom he knows personally, and who is prepared to work with him on my case. Dr. Richard Fried has considerable experience with cancer patients, and has offered to be Lenny's mentor, both in this treatment with me, and other aspects of anthroposophic medicine that Lenny wishes to develop in tandem with his own expertise in homeopathy. He feels this might be more productive than both of us needing to build a relationship with someone we don't know. While seeing Dr. Fried, I can also work with a curative eurythmist, for eurythmy is one of the chief supporting therapies.

Though I certainly hadn't calculated on further travels, this seems to be a time for going with the flow – even the somewhat alarming cash flow – into which this illness is sweeping me. So, I agree. I particularly want to begin eurythmy as soon as possible. Though I don't believe the Druids performed it, it is a potent and necessary adjunct to the mistletoe therapy.

Eurythmy is a form of movement expressing in space the world of formative forces out of which we were created and through which we are continually enlivened and maintained. It is performed artistically and taught in groups, as a generally revitalizing individual and social experience. It is an integral part of the Waldorf curriculum, indirectly educating many physical and mental capacities.

Curative eurythmy is the therapeutic application of certain movements and gestures which activate forces within the body so they can heal what has gone awry. It could be called "immune-therapy", and calls strongly upon the etheric body which, as we have seen, is the healer, repairing and regenerating areas that the astral body has assaulted and destroyed. As one doctor put it: stress on the astral body has caused it to press too deeply into the etheric, breaking the latter up into independent areas of life-activity (tumors), and treatment must "glue" the etheric back again, so that the Ego, which contains the blueprint for the organism, can enter these areas again and imprint the proper design upon them.

Though I had done eurythmy in a group, I had never had curative eurythmy before. This must be prescribed by a doctor. The movements work quite directly and powerfully into organs and body systems and must be carefully monitored. I was certainly interested in experiencing this, particularly if it could do the trick of glueing me back together again!

I've only been to Pennsylvania once before, when the corn stood high in the Amish farm fields, and we lay luxuriously beside a friend's swimming pool in between sessions of a workshop we held on our way to live in Detroit. I wondered what this winter trip would hold for me. I call this friend, with whom I've vaguely kept in touch over the intervening years. Not strongly in touch, however, for almost her first words on hearing why I am coming are:

"Oh, I had a mastectomy myself two years ago." How I wish I'd known, and is this already one reason for my visit – to re-establish contact with Suzanne again?

"Which breast was yours?" she asks.

"Left."

"Oh, you can't join the New Age Amazons then. We only allow Right Breasts into our club!"

"But I thought I *was* an Amazon. Didn't they cut their left breasts off?"

"Think!" Says Suzanne. "Which side would *you* loose an arrow from?" Wrong again! Maybe I'm a left-handed Amazon – trust me!

We fly over a quiet winter landscape to Philadelphia, landing in such a peculiar and terrifying fashion that I realize I am afraid of dying, however glibly I speak of my demise. The limousine drives me along gentle, wood-fringed roads, which curve here, and go up and down. What a delight after the flat, graph-paper system of Metro Detroit. And what a delight to see Suzanne again, have Mexican food together, and catch up on times spent apart, yet not in such a dissimilar fashion, inwardly at least. So we grow.

Next day, another friend picks me up in a blizzard and drives me to Dr. Fried's office beside a defunct train station, the tracks already piled high with drifting snow. He is a slim man, younger than me, with an aura of quietly concentrated energy, and a gaze that doesn't miss much. He asks me some interesting questions – interesting because they are so different from any conventional physicians ask – and examines the palms of my hands.

"Do you have eczema?" He enquires politely.

"No. I cut my fingers instead of the garlic, with my chopping knife."

"Ah," he says, significantly. It probably *is* significant, too; as everything and anything about me might be.

He also asks politely if I would mind his examining my breast, which he does with a delicate, professional touch, and waits while I pull my clothes about me again. How different it feels to have such an interview properly dressed, instead of clutching a ridiculous scrap of paper towel round meters of naked flesh.

We talk some more and, to my great pleasure, he tells me that while he doesn't usually recommend treatments – feeling the patient must choose – he does wonder if radiation is the best choice for me. He also thinks I am an excellent candidate for *Iscador*.

"Do you mind changing to *Iscador*?" He adds. "You've been taking *Abnoba*, another brand.

"I guess I never thought about it. Is there a difference?"

"Mainly in people's preference. I'm familiar with *Iscador* myself. Some patients feel a particular attachment to one or the other." *Iscador* is the name I always knew, together with all the people who had taken it. I clearly had faith in it. "Thy faith has made thee whole." Yes, I feel happy with *Iscador*. Dr. Fried gives me the address of Hiscia, in Switzerland, from which I can order some.

He adds to my pharmocopoeia; copper, to be followed by homeopathic iron; belladonna; *stibium* (another name for antimony, which Basil Valentinus, the alchemist, once described as one of the seven wonders of the world.). These lovely evocative names are inscribed on cozy brown bottles, with special stoppers that release what looks like clear water in rhythmic drops – here 20, here 15, – usually to be taken before meals. He prescribes fever baths and mentions coffee enemas but, reading my expression quickly, tells me colonics would be the next best thing. There's only one appropriate orifice for coffee, as far as I'm concerned.

Because I'm familiar with anthroposophical jargon, he mentions that a chief problem is my "hypertrophied astral body". I always thought hypertrophied would describe worn-out elastic; flabby, shrivelled, that can only really be thrown away. But I guess – or hope – that Dr. Fried has something else in mind for my astral body. I'm not ready to discard it yet, for all the trouble it causes me!

Well, we seem to have taken care of my body, or bodies, but our session doesn't end there. Dr. Fried gives me a sudden penetrating look.
"What's your meditation life like?" He asks.
Oh, blast! Can he tell that easily? Try as I might, and do, meditation is terrifically hard for me. I seldom seem to reach the point where it become the nourishing force that others claim for it. I tell him this. No point in lying. Besides, from his sympathetic nod, it's clear he's deduced this – probably from the state of my fingertips!
"If you could try," he says, "for at least fifteen minutes a day, I think that would be very good for you." I know it would. As good as a dozen brown bottles of medicines.

He shakes my hand warmly when we part. And, despite the shame I feel about my spiritual inadequacy, I leave his office encouraged and affirmed.

Across his parking lot is a small white cottage in which Alice, the curative eurythmist, lives. I visit her next. Her space has a quiet peacefulness that is quite tangible, filled with soft colors, and Alice's own calm and vital attentiveness. Her rich voice guides me gently through some pretty bizarre movements and, though I wobble wildly with one leg in the air, I feel increasingly suffused with a steadying power that both she and the exercises evoke in me. Later, I lie under a woven, pure wool blanket, feeling a stirring of warm currents within my body. "Try to let your mind free when you rest your body. Your mind must rest too. That's very important." Lying under a woolly rug, resting my addled brain, quite regenerated after a few minutes of these apparently negligible movements, is what I call healing.

"Your body needs to remember movements it made long long ago," says Alice softly. "The body was formed out of these living gestures, and is sustained by them. Do eurythmy with love. Enjoy it."

I breathe deeply. I feel an ache of sadness for breaking faith with these subtle energies out of which I sprang, which still carry me, and whose forms and rhythms I have so violated. Would I have re-membered such realities if I had not fallen sick?

Back in Detroit, it is instantly clear to me that I do not want radiation at this stage. Statistics, opinions, even my own fears, have played their part in this choice. It is, however, the haunting experience of those few moments of eurythmy that finally decides me. I cannot do further violence to those living, weaving forces. I must hereafter learn to nourish them, or give them the opportunity to nourish me.

Chapter 9

DIET

"First know food. From food all things are born, by food they live, toward food they move, into food they return."
— Upanishads.

"'We won't find the diet too hard, Judge.' Don't you loathe it when doctors use the word "we" when it applies only and solely to yourself. He could go home and gobble fifty biscuits and ten baked Alaskas ... while me, I'm starving on a diet, so I meditated in a furious way."
— Clock Without Hands, Carson McCullors.

Diet – that's a big one. The big D. to beat the Big C! Holistic pundits have stressed diet for a long time and many consider it *the* cure for cancer as well as a host of other diseases. Even the orthodox medical community somewhat belatedly acknowledge that a faulty diet may play a part in the advent of cancer and display bright posters full of leafy vegetables on their office walls. That it might play a role in a person's recovery "has not yet been conclusively proved" to quote one oncologist; a fairly astonishing comment in the light of growing evidence that it does; even in the light of logic to which I always imagined the sciences were heavily pledged. If what you eat may land you in one place, surely what you eat next may bring you out again. To what absurd levels of unreality has modern man descended when the connection between food and health has been severed in our minds!

Of course diet may not heal us, just as living exclusively on junk food may not catalyze a situation in which cancer can occur. But once one has cancer a good diet can certainly contribute mightily to helping the body regain the forces it needs to fight this disease. Apart from the actual intake of certain substances which, hopefully, revitalize the body, going on a diet is a tremendous act of will. This in itself is a healing deed. As we've seen, cancer occurs in those places where we have, so to speak, lost control and connection. By turning our attention towards our own flesh, by the rigorous discipline required to follow any dietary regime, we inevitably regain some mastery over ourselves.

Diet was therefore one of my own most basic therapies. It also became one of the most challenging areas of my life. It faced me with choices and, as my son once ruefully reflected: "Choices are the worst thing about being alive. I wish we didn't have to make them all the time." How I agreed with him!

I began with the diet outlined by anthroposophic medicine, but almost every day I was offered alternatives – each promising better and yet better results, and backing up their claims so vividly that from time to time I felt I might die of pure fright, not cancer, as I learned about lifelong deprivations of vitamins, minerals and many substances I'd never heard of before. I wondered how I had walked the earth so many years, clearly lacking just about everything I needed in order to do so. And I was frequently tempted to clear my fridge of all the wholesome ingredients I had just brought home to replace them with others that were said to be more wholesome yet. What made it worse were the deeply conflicting opinions. One regime hinted at immortality on a daily dose of raw beet juice. Another declared that beets must be avoided at all costs!

Perhaps the most rigorous diet I came across is that developed by Dr. Max Gerson, *A Cancer Therapy: The Result of Fifty Cases*. This is based on completely de-toxifying and rebuilding the body, mainly with combinations of raw vegetable juice. It requires an almost complete withdrawal from life for about eighteen months, since it takes all one's time – with help from others – to prepare the juices hourly in low-tech ways, drink them, clean up, take a coffee enema, and begin all over again. However there have been some astonishing cures in extreme cases, documented in his book. Beata Bishop, in her own fine and moving account, *My Triumph Over Cancer*, records her process of healing (melanoma) and rejuvenation in ways that astounded her, as well as others. I rejected this diet because it was far too demanding. The thought of interrupting my life with Adam every four hours for a coffee enema did not bear thinking about! But I was, and still am, glad to know of it. It's good to have some hot options in hand, in case I need to use them one day.

I did, however, add raw vegetable juices to my own diet. They bring much needed vitamins directly into the system and impose no strain on the digestive system. The right combinations can taste delicious. Carrot juice is the well-known favorite. Other juice cures stress its importance. It has an added charm since it gradually suffuses your skin with a golden glow that people mistake for a trip to Florida. I quickly became addicted to my daily dose and at least looked a great deal healthier than many members of the medical community attempting to heal me!

Perhaps the hot favorite in diets is macrobiotics. An excellent personal account of healing through this diet is given by Dr. Anthony Sattilaro in his book *Recalled by Life*. Despite his initial skepticism, stemming from his own conventional medical background, Dr. Sattilaro turned around his own extensive cancer and describes the process of his own conversion and healing quite compellingly. Besides this book, I read or heard of so many cures for cancer as well as a host of other ailments that it seemed foolhardy to reject this path. However, I found it was one I could not take. Whenever I tried it I felt what I can only describe as a kind of "inner darkening". It is not simply that I dislike large slimy leaves of seaweed or have for years been a strict member of the "No-Tofu" brigade. When I travelled in Japan I thoroughly enjoyed the food. But it does not fit me here, or now. In the same way that I have never been attracted to take up an Eastern spiritual path, while having respect for such disciplines, I seek something that has its sources in the west at this point of my life. Turning eastward felt like a return and I needed to go forward now.

Actually, macrobiotics has as one of its principles the emphasis on eating substances that are grown locally and there are few Umeboshi plum trees and little seaweed in south east Michigan! Not many rice paddies either, of course, but I can live with the fact that I do eat vast quantities of brown rice. I do, however, resonate to the idea of eating local produce wherever possible. Not only is it much fresher, it is also a way of re-inserting ourselves into the community of root, leaf and blossom that surrounds and sustains us. Cancer is such an image of falling out and away from natural processes. Perhaps what I was fumbling towards in those early days was a form of western macrobiotics. Its general principles feel sound to me if they could be translated into a quite different context and culture.

Another golden rule of this system is to seek a balance of foods within any meal. This is described as a balance between *yang* and *yin*. Available literature can amplify this better than I can, though I know sadly that it is not as Cynthia wickedly suggests simply a matter of following a large steak (*yang*) with a rich, sugary dessert (*yin*). However, a balance of substances within each meal makes sense, and should include a harmony of color, texture and taste – as any good chef knows.

Then there is the whole attitude to food. Each meal should be prepared and eaten with devotion – a celebration of one's community with the earth and dependence upon it. Penny Brohn, in her book, *The Bristol Programme* – (not, I believe, yet published in this country,) quotes a healthy old man whose diet was not impeccable, as saying: "It's not what you eat, but what you think while you're eating it." I think there is great truth in that, and it is certainly easier to think good thoughts while eating a meal that has been reverently prepared than while hastily inhaling a Big Mac and french fries. (Though I do feel something akin to a religious fervor when offered a certain brand of Swiss chocolate; not yet, to my knowledge, included on any cancer diet sheet!)

Besides these two major dietary cures, there were several lesser ones, and I frequently wondered if I should change course. But the anthroposophic diet felt right for me, and as I turned away from more restrictive regimes, I argued happily that butter (so notably missing from other diet sheets) might even have a positive alchemical conjunction with eurythmy and *Iscador*!

Besides inspiring a new medical approach, Rudolf Steiner also helped develop what is known as biodynamic agriculture, (a heightened form of organic farming and gardening.) This is practised throughout the world. Nutrition – one bridge between medicine and agriculture – is considered a high priority for all. Once you have cancer it becomes an imperative. (A good small booklet describing the cancer diet is *Cancer & Nutrition* by Dr. Gerhard Schmidt –

available in most health food stores.) Apart from the faith I have in the whole approach of anthroposophy, what I particularly like are the explanations and images of the value of each food or food group. I find it much easier to take on board an unfamiliar substance if I can actively imagine what it is bringing me.

A high proportion of a variety of organic whole grains is recommended. (There is actually a grain for each day of the week which can be fun to try once in a while.) The seed of a plant is full of "sun-forces" and thus grains bring sun into the organism. Here we have the image of light and warmth again, which the cancer-afflicted body so urgently needs. It also requires an effort on the part of the body to digest grains and this work in itself is strengthening. Much more effort is required to assimilate plants than animal products, since we are closer to animals ourselves. We grow slack, lazy and weak if we eat a lot of meat. Now we have to wrest the proteins out of the grains rather than being handed them straight on a plate. This is, in fact, a pretty low protein diet – not more, so Lenny told me, than around 20 grams a day.

While ideally all food should be biodynamically grown, the next best thing is organic and locally produced. No packaged, canned, frozen or chemically treated foods are recommended. One is seeking foods which still retain their life forces, which modern agricultural and commercial procedures have effectively destroyed. I was amazed when moving to this country to see how many products first had everything they owned naturally removed, or destroyed and then re-introduced artificially. Milk is happily pasteurized and homogenized, for instance, and then advertised as containing added vitamins A and D! I was thrilled to find one company selling "Milk – Just Milk", but it went out of business shortly afterwards. "Just Milk" is clearly not a seller for the average American!

As vegetables should be fresh and cooked in ways that retain their value, fruits – also organic – should be sun-ripened. No more bunches of green bananas left to grow yellow and brown in your fruit bowl. Actually, organic bananas are quite hard to find and, as with other fruit, seldom look as appetizing as their chemically-aided counterparts. This is true of much organic produce, but it is simply that we've forgotten how things were a few decades ago, and that looks aren't everything! I rediscovered a part of my forgotten childhood, finding bugs and maggots at the heart of things. I recalled the particular gesture my mother used when she was discreetly removing baked caterpillars from our cabbage or broccoli. As I dealt with these various home owners again, I consoled myself with the thought that their presence probably confirmed the nutritiousness of the plant. If a bug is not attracted, or can survive on one, it probably has little to offer us!

I further learned, from my politically conscious friends that if we cannot get everything organically grown we should at least avoid anything that comes from those countries – mainly Central and South American – in which North America has a vested interest. Apparently we supply them with many chemicals and fertilizers that are banned here and then buy in – to sell at high profit – produce grown by those means.

Where the anthroposophical diet breaks with some others is its inclusion of fats. These should, however, be as pure as possible. Good quality oils, fresh untreated butter and soft cheeses are allowed. The purpose of these is to build warmth back into the organism. Lenny told me that butter has a melting temperature of 98.4°, expressing in this way a quite intimate connection with the human organism. Good quality yoghourt is also a staple. It contains whatever is needed to introduce healthy bacteria into the intestinal tract – what one nutritionalist I met called "the good fairies" who deal with the whole process of assimilation of food and the distribution of energies acquired from it.

An interesting addition to, or subtraction from, many other diets is anything cold or iced. There is such an emphasis on building warmth back into the organism. So farewell ice cream and thirty ice cubes in every glass of water. For a Britisher reared on the lukewarm – beer included – this posed no hardship for me. Iced drinks always make my eyes hurt anyway, and in this country there always seems to be more ice than drink! I could imagine this deprivation would be pretty tough for most Americans who must eat more ice cream and drink more freezing drinks than any other nation in the world.

The Great No-Nos that I have not found stressed elsewhere are those plants of the nightshade family: potatoes, tomatoes, peppers and eggplant. (The Max Gerson diet actually depends highly on the first two, used in a soup claimed to have been invented by Hippocrates.) The reason for omitting them is that they themselves grow in a somewhat tumorous way. I learned later that, if one really cannot resist tomatoes, one should at least avoid them while on a cycle of *Iscador*. It is actually quite hard to avoid them. It is amazing to notice what a fundamental part they play in the American cuisine. Mushrooms are also taboo. If one honestly contemplates the life-style of a mushroom, springing up in the darkness on such unseemly soil – as does cancer – it is hard to relish one thereafter. I am also amazed at what a frequent addition mushrooms are in vegetarian meals. At my local health food restaurant I can barely find a dish or sauce that excludes them.

Having decided more or less what one is going to eat the next challenge is getting hold of it. I had great momentary yearnings to abandon my life in the Detroit area and seek a home on a biodynamic farm. My nearest source of biodynamic vegetables was in Canada – a six-hour journey – and I was extremely grateful to our Christian Community priest and his wife who frequently lugged bushels of carrots and beets back with them when they visited Toronto. They once delivered these to my door, tied up in a red ribbon – perhaps my best Christmas present this year!

I found myself spending most of my days racing all over town in search of one or other perfect ingredient, and hoping I would have time left to prepare the food I had acquired. (I also had to cater to Adam and his friends. Though I may be guilty of systematically poisoning them, they were not about to accept millet patties in exchange for spaghetti or pizza. As Adam commented drily, observing my plate one day: "If you don't watch out you'll turn into one of the Waldorf-

Nutrifood people, with their shaggy hair and craggy clothes and those awful clumpy sandals." It was no good pointing out to him that most of the people we knew who were associated with the Waldorf School and shopped at Nutrifoods did not fit this category. I knew what he meant. And even if I became shaggier and craggier over the next few years, I felt I owed it to him to keep our home and what we offered here within socially acceptable limits!) So I was kept pretty busy, fulfilling our different needs and it was when I realized I was devoting the same kind of nervous, frantic energy to healing myself that had probably led to my getting sick in the first place, that I decided I would have to rethink and reorganize. I had hardly time to actually eat. I almost never sat down to relax over my glass of fresh juice. I also frequently questioned the point of juicing carrots in order to keep alive long enough to be able to juice some more. This hardly seemed a fulfilling destiny! I decided I had to compromise.

We all have stratagems for survival and mine were as follows. I decided I would allot a certain amount of time for shopping, minimizing driving as much as possible. I sensed that hunching tensely over the wheel on a crowded freeway was not particularly healing, and I felt the impact of driving more deeply than I had before surgery. This would leave time for preparing and even eating my food in a more leisurely fashion. It might even leave time for some other activities! Then I decided I would believe that what I was eating was doing me good, even if I broke here and there with the purists. While I may be accused of gross self-deception, this felt necessary to me.

As soon as I did decide this, helpful affirmations arrived. Mary-Jo told me that most chemicals get caught in the fibers of plants when juiced and seldom actually reach the juice itself. Thus I felt justified in using fresh local produce that may have been sprinkled with pesticides, in the hope that the sprinkles were not reaching me. The Max Gersonites are not permitted high-tech juicers, but labor with old-fashioned gadgets, pressing juice through cheesecloth, etc., all of which clearly retains vitamins and minerals in their purest and most potent forms. I rejected this in favor of a centrifugal juicer and not even the most highly recommended kind. This – the Champion – had such a large bullying presence that I felt I'd always live in fear of it, have dark nightmares of it leaping off its pedestal and chomping everything in sight. I chose a reasonably priced elegant little Swiss machine that may be marginally less effective but produces a stream of green and red vitamins in the quiet and orderly manner for which the Swiss are renowned.

The decision to settle for some produce that was not classified as organic became firmer as winter progressed. Apart from my Canadian carrots, local organic ones developed a rusty taste that I mistrusted as well as thoroughly disliked. Their appearance was hardly seductive either. (I was reminded of a rather wicked entry I and my fellow author made about the condition of vegetables at a macrobiotic London restaurant when we were writing a health food guide in the early days of seeds and sprouts. To our astonishment and dismay our publisher insisted on sending the proprietor a copy for his approval. His response was unequivocal, suggesting I stick his so-called "shrivelled carrots" up my fat journalistic ass! I promptly replied that his carrots looked as though they had already been used in this way, and commented that his wrath was hardly compatible with the *yin* personality (meek and passive) that he had been at pains to impress upon me in our interview was a direct consequence of the diet he followed and offered his customers. After a delightful blazing interchange we actually became friends, but he never convinced me that months-old limp and puckered carrots, however virtuously grown, are superior to those that are freshly plucked.)

Another friend gave me a soap product alleged to remove all surface chemicals. I began to use this in good faith, reminding myself that by spring I could grow my own veggies and help Lulu and Al in their latest enterprise – a five-acre farm by Lake Huron – in return for some harvesting. In the spring I talked to suppliers in my local Farmers' Market and found two or three who only used pesticides in an emergency and fertilized with their own farm manure. I often felt their fruit and vegetables, picked that very morning on Michigan farms, and often replete with small green caterpillars, were a much better deal than a limp, fully organic lettuce that had been flown in from California a week before. We all know what plane trips do to our life-forces. I doubt a lettuce can withstand the experience any better than we can.

I grew to love the shapes, textures and colors of carrot, parsley, spinach and kale. I would find myself lost in contemplation of their singular beauty; crenellated leaf and sturdy root. The colors seemed twice as vivid as any I had seen before, even before sousing them in the special soap. When I did get good organic ones they were an exquisite luxury. I would feel almost decadent sitting down to relish a sumptuous dish of spinach, green onion, carrot and beet. I would recall past pleasures; all those lobster claws and quivering cream and liqueur desserts I'd glutted myself upon as a London debutante. They no longer appealed. Millet and buckwheat simmered in garlic and tamari were now house specialties that could hardly be bettered by more lavish fare. I felt I was well and truly on my way; grains and veggies, Amish butter, colorful salads, homemade granola full of amaranth, (the power grain of the Aztecs,) vine-ripened raisins, Hunza apricots, washed down with mint or linden flower tea.

Of course there were moments of regression and acute desire. It was as if two voices spoke in me. One, strident and raucous, demanded coffee, slabs of chocolate, whipped cream. The other meekly requested: "If you don't mind, I'd like an orange please." I began to listen to this second voice. I imagined it came from my liver, now tentatively encouraged to believe I might listen to it after so many deaf years. Lenny told me our livers actually taste food from the moment we think of eating it and the chief tragedy for this organ is that we feed it substances that are quite foreign to it, that it cannot recognize and therefore assimilate. He added, interestingly, that microwave systems cause the cells in food to reverse direction so the liver is totally confused and he attributes the increase in liver cancer to the extensive use of them. Though I have always intuitively rejected microwave, I still imagined my liver in a constant anxiety state, as I used to be at boarding school, awaiting the dreaded aroma on tapioca days. I began to enjoy cossetting and reassuring it.

I did strike bargains from time to time. Life is all about the imperfect and the compromise! On many afternoons I ceremonially made myself a cup of organically grown coffee (Cafe Altura), freshly ground, topped with cream and bottomed with a teaspoon of sugar. I sat out on my back porch and drank this with relish, accompanied by a cigarette smoked in a transparent filter invented by an Italian, which purports to restrain 70% of the carcinogens. If I felt guilty, I would follow this soon after with a tumbler of carrot juice. If I resented feeling guilty, I would remind my liver that I had treated it to massage recently – plus, what about the colonics I was paying for on its behalf?

Colonics were the other end of the spectrum, so to speak. It is not merely a matter of what we put into ourselves, but what comes out again. Cancer invariably occurs in a body system with a high level of toxicity, so cleansing that system is a high priority. The noxious residues of even the purest foods must be eliminated with all possible speed. Colonics are one way of effecting this – the way I chose as a creative compromise between nothing, and the coffee enemas I was not prepared to give myself.

Even these began as an ordeal to which no self-respecting, properly inhibited Britisher would gladly submit. I recalled my days at an all-girls' boarding school, lining up after breakfast for syrup-of-figs, failure writ large upon those of us who had not had a "movement" for three days. "Keep your bowels open and your mouth shut," was the high injunction, maybe even invisibly inscribed over the sacred portals of that bleak brick institute, as the Greek temples carried the command: "Man Know Thyself." After the first occasion, I felt irrationally angry, fantasizing all kinds of unhygienic practices on the part of my nutritional therapist. Were the fixtures properly sterilized? Would I come here to cure cancer and contract AIDS? What a tatty rug she has too. "What's more, if she asks me how I feel, I won't tell her", I resolve, waking at night filled with illimitable rage. So I discover – at least by American standards – that I'm anal-retentive, along with all my other neuroses.

But I persevere and the experience improves. I don't notice any particular effect and never know if this therapy has been unsuccessful or that I may simply be insensitive to its subtleties. Still – going for a weekly colonic is another act of will.

It is this therapist who gently guides my awareness into another awesome dimension of diet: food combinations – not just what you eat, but with what else and when. Typically I balk initially. This is too much to take on board, having already set sail. Cheri is patient, as I am not.

"Take it step by step," she counsels, while I irritably grapple with my constitutional desire to reach *Nirvana* in one stride. She takes no offence when I turn down her offers of enzymes, freeze-dried carrot patties and other nutritious tidbits she brings to her office every week. I do accept *Rejuvelac*: a brackish-tasting water drained from fermented wheatberries, said to be full of chlorophyll – something else cancer cells can't abide. But it often stands forgotten in my fridge. Adam drank some once, mistaking it for vanilla pop. His expression captured my own feelings when I did remember to gulp some down.

One week I bring home a medium size bag of sprouts I ordered, having imagined them as little juicy green shoots. They were actually raw beans and lentils, indeed modestly sprouting, but I was meant to eat them whole. I put handfuls in salads, particularly when friends were coming to supper, and kept this up gallantly for a week. The bag never seemed to grow lighter. It had a peculiar magical ability to replenish itself. To reduce the amount felt like a heroic task so beloved of myth and fairy tale. One day I, or my unconscious, allowed the bag to spill. I spent fifteen minutes sweeping up piles of dusty pulses from my kitchen floor but when I picked up the bag itself it felt as full as ever. I emptied it on my compost. Enough was enough. They could return to me in another season, another form!

Apart from wondering if a daily dose of Drāno wouldn't solve all problems, I continue with colonics and am slowly but surely converted to food combinations over the following weeks. When Cheri vividly described the consequences of a piece of fruit travelling in tandem with protein through my digestive system, I realized I could not henceforth allow such things to occur.

"Protein takes eight hours to digest. Fruit only twenty minutes. So the fruit must wait – let's see – seven hours and forty minutes for the protein to be ready to travel on. In that time, you may imagine the state of the fruit!" Indeed, I could imagine it. Addled, fermented, emitting toxic fumes with which accidents at Three Mile Island hardly compare. I've marched on pollution issues, written my senator frequently about chemical waste. Was I to permit this within my own flesh? Clearly not. So I began to learn all over again. And it was really far simpler than I first supposed. No protein after two o'clock, fruit always eaten at a separate meal and, wherever possible, combining things marked "good" and avoiding things marked "poor" on a little chart Cheri gave me and which I tacked up on my wall.

When Marjanna wrote plaintively: "but what about the olive – is it fruit or vegetable?" I replied that I thought – if fruit – there had to be exceptions to every rule. We all have to have something to live for, after all. And if, for Marjanna, olives are one of those things I am sure she stands a higher chance of survival if she can happily write them into next week's menus, combining them with whatever she pleases, and eating them with joy and confidence.

I remind myself of Lenny's injunction: "Enjoy your food. Your life too. Fanaticism is dangerous." And I recall a comment of Dr. Steiner himself: "It is better to eat meat than think meat." Though I do not believe he addressed this to a cancer patient, I interpret this to mean that if I am going to be driven to nightly frenzies of desire for some delicacy that is taboo, it may be to my advantage spiritually if I indulge myself, whatever havoc it wreaks upon my flesh!

Chapter 10

FEVER BATHS AND OTHER DELIGHTS

"The time has come," the Walrus said
To talk of other things:
Of shoes – and ships – and sealing wax –
And cabbages – and kings –
And why the sea is boiling hot –
And whether pigs have wings."
           – Alice in Wonderland, Lewis Carroll.

Adam and I have just had a blazing row. He stampedes upstairs, yelling imprecations, and wisely slams his door. I am left to stew in my own juice. It is clearly a good time to take my first fever bath.

I go through my checklist and begin by making a pot of linden flower tea. Apparently this loosens the connective tissues. I drank a lot of it in pregnancy. I am now directed to do so after my bath. It should be as hot as I can bear it when I get in, and I must gradually add more hot water and soak there until I've got my temperature up a few degrees. No-one has told me how high this should go, since Dr. Fried assumed that Dorothea would monitor me, and she and I decided I could probably do as good a job, if amateur, myself. It seemed complicated for me to take a bath in her house, with five small children rushing about, and I'd eventually have the journey home. Here, I can simply stay cozy and fall asleep.

When the bath is ready, I slowly lower myself into it. It is hot! I begin to turn quite pink. Remembering baths in Japan at various hot-spring spas, I knew the best technique is to stay as still as possible. You don't feel the heat quite as much; it gives the experience a somewhat dreamlike quality. Emboldened, I add more hot water, feeling my scalp prickle and my eyes cloud with sweat. After a few minutes, I take my temperature. It has only risen a few points. To keep heat in, I try to submerge my whole body. Baths are not designed for this; only a midget could get both halves in. Assuming a sort of recumbent lotus position, I do the best I can. I make sure that at least my breasts are covered, add more water and wait. After ten minutes or so I can really feel something happening. My heart is pounding wildly, sweat is now streaming down my head and face, I have a rather scary sense I might dissolve. I poke out my arm for the thermometer. It still barely reads 100 degrees. I take a deep breath and try again.

For the next five minutes or so, I'm engaged in a tremendous battle of wills. My body clamors to leap up and out. It knows what's best for it, and right now that would be to dash straight into a blizzard. But I hold it back tenaciously, fighting for control, feeling increasingly dissolute, dizzy and out-of-breath. At last I can bear it no longer. I stagger up, dry myself hurriedly – the air feels freezing – and totter to my room, curling up under towels, a down comforter and two thick wool blankets. Only then do I take my temperature again. Oh, triumph! It reads 102.8°! Now I must lie here for an hour or so, letting the fever run its course while I sip linden flower tea.

About fifteen minutes later, Adam comes in. I am drenched in sweat. My hair is standing up on end around my crimson, throbbing face. He takes one look at me – a look I shall never forget – and enquires acidly:

"And what do the *other* kids do when *their* Moms are taking fever baths?"

What, indeed? I may one day find out. Unless, as Adam's tone implied, no other mother would indulge in such eccentric practices. But, seeing him, and imagining him seeing me, I begin to giggle and, when I've got enough breath, suggest it's the ideal time for us to play a game of Scrabble.

So that's what we do. It becomes our Sunday evening ritual. I recommend it, if there are by chance other mothers out there. You only have to poke a finger out once in a while to juggle your letters about. You can't think straight, so your words are usually simple, muddled, or drawn from a world of fantasy. This means your child will invariably win – a guaranteed satisfaction to him or her, which may not be theirs in other games. And, of course you are in no state to mind losing yourself. There's no self to lose, for at least a couple of hours, and then it's time for lights out and goodnight.

I tried visualization. Like diet, its exponents claim it as the ultimate heal-all. I do not deride it, for many of the claims are clearly justified. My godson, who suffered for years with an inoperable brain tumor, often eased the pressure by imaging the tumor as a lettuce that a rabbit would munch up. Others have clearly activated healing powers that have reduced or completely exterminated their cancers. I simply found it extremely hard to do, often with as little experienced effect as my bouts with meditation bring. I suppose they vaguely belong in the same category. I feel quite some shame, owning my incapacity. I sincerely believe in the power of imaging, use it in my own practice, and evoke images for myself quite frequently. Perhaps in the innumerable choices offered us when we set about this business of healing, visualization was less alluring than others. One can't eat everything on a menu without winding up feeling sick.

I read the Simonton's book – *Getting Well Again*. I had heard Carl Simonton speak the previous year, and have a boundless admiration for his work. So I begin following the procedures outlined. I have a hard time getting aggressive images for my white blood cells and learn that, on top of all my other defects, I'm clearly too passive, and just the type to let the cancer take over entirely. When I firmly place pictures of sharks raring to dine on my cancer cells, they turn into technicolor images from Jaws, and don't stop at the cancer, but happily munch my breasts, nipples and all. I swear I actually saw one wink at me! I wind up getting the giggles. I've often felt my psyche was peopled by script writers for the Marx Brothers, and here they come again.

When I do manage to find images that I think are a fair compromise between the recommended aggressiveness and my own more moderate preferences, I simply feel extremely bored. Nor am I suffused with the promised light and energy. These I receive abundantly when I take the Christian sacrament, spend time in the company of friends, or watch a scarlet cardinal alight in the snowy branches of my apple tree.

*   *   *

Another activity is literally *activity* – i.e. exercise. No-one is in this game for long before discovering some people have put their cancer into remission simply through jogging. They've continued – so far as I know – on junk food, old habits, no visualization. They've simply run their cancer off, or outrun it, so to speak. Penny Brohn, along with all her other therapies, swam sixty-four lengths in her local swimming baths and lives to tell the tale, and recommend exercise as a vital ingredient in one's recovery plan. I was too shy to go swimming at the YMCA that first winter, with my angry red scar and lopsided arms. I also suspected that, even were I brave enough to parade my mutilations, I would most likely drown. It's quite hard enough for me to keep afloat when all my limbs are in working order. I didn't fancy jogging. The solution arrived in the form of a Rebounder – a dandy little circular trampoline which I purchased for under $20 along with some encouraging literature. The most encouraging statement was that rebounding for as little as three minutes was extremely effective in activating the immune-system and beginning to clear the lymph. These days I'm all for activities that only last three minutes!

I discover too around this time a delightful little book – *God Helps Those Who Help Themselves* by Hanna Kroeger. Apart from recommending such things as going to bed and keeping warm if you feel a cold coming on, she gives valuable tips on how to concoct quick simple home brews for a number of ailments. It is from her that I learn that cucumber juice is excellent for cleansing the lymph system, so it seems appropriate to swig some before leaping about. This I do for a while until I realize my juicer can't handle cucumbers. At least I'm certain they were what caused the gadget to go into a wild frenzied tribal dance, shuddering and juddering all over the tabletop. When finally brought to rest it revealed its cannibalism. It had devoured large sections of its own interior and I was left with a glass of juiced plastic. Since this happened with two replacements whenever I mixed cucumbers with my daily dose of carrots, I had to abandon it. But for a while I have some extremely satisfying sessions, pounding and gurgling juicily up and down. It was a quite painless form of exercise. I bounced till I began to prickle vaguely all over, feeling the warmth eventually reach my fingertips. This happened long before my legs gave out. When I watched joggers pounding the pavement, I felt no envy. My springy little sessions were far preferable.

It is while springing merrily one day that I have a brainwave. Surely this is the time and place to do my visualizing – two for the price of one! And now I can find images that really suit. I picture my lymph as a light-filled juicy sap, racing through my system, clearing out debris. My cancer cells are simply washed away in this energizing spring tide. By the time my toes and fingers tingle I can even believe, however physiologically inaccurate, that the malignant cells are dropping off my extremities. A wholly delightful experience I try to give myself each day.

*   *   *

Another therapy is painting – or, more accurately, working with color through the medium of paint. The artistic therapies are a fundamental part of anthroposophical healing and, as with all therapies, designed to work very precisely upon specific imbalances.

Painting is particularly effective in regulating the astral body and harmonizing it with the etheric forces again. As we have seen, the astral body is destructive, continually eroding and consuming the etheric body in the service of consciousness. One can generally see the effects of an over-active astral body in thinner, more nervy types. There is a tendency to too much form and consciousness. (By contrast, dreamier types, whose bodies may burgeon more shapelessly, will work in clay to discipline the unconscious vitality of the etheric.) An illustration of these two types – sometimes referred to as "nerve-sense" and "metabolic" respectively – in the animal kingdom would be the bird and the cow: the first bright-eyed, pecking things to pieces, the second lazily chewing the cud!

It is interesting that my own cancer was discovered in a calcified area, rather than a burgeoning tumor; striking evidence of my own tendency to harden and crystallize rather than flow with vitality. This further illustrates Steiner's formulation of the polarity between the nerve-sense cephalic pole, with its cold hardening tendencies and the metabolic-limb system, full of warmth and activity, between which the rhythmic circulatory system mediates as the great balancer. All the artistic therapies introduce rhythm in one way or another, as a breathing process between the patient and the substance or activity in which he or she is engaged. Painting, however, was clearly the therapy for me. As soon as I had time and energy, I called my friend and teacher, Eve, and fixed a session with her at her home about fifteen minutes away.

"Green, I think", says Eve, staring into the middle distance. "Red and green." Yes, I think so too. These are the colors I feel I need.
"Green for healing. Red at the center, green at the periphery. Would that be the one?"
Yes, that's it. The meditation in two colors that Steiner described as the breathing exercise for today – the new yoga – working with colors on a page that in turn work back on the breath, the rhythm between heart and lung.

So I begin. It's been a long time. Standing at arm's length before the easel, the large white page, I feel afraid. The journey about to start will be a painful journey of self-discovery. As I build the color layer upon layer, my inner world of doubt, confusion, rigidity will be unpeeling like onion skins. My first strokes are pale and tentative. Every time is new, as unknown as the first.

I've been painting with Eve fairly regularly for several years. I met her soon after my arrival here and we formed an instant bond. Since I had just had exploratory surgery for heavy menstrual bleeding, it seemed natural to ask her if artistic therapy might help, rather than the hysterectomy or hormone therapy I knew would be recommended next. Even if it didn't, I wanted to paint. I wanted to know Eve better. We clearly had some deep and mysterious connection that even others acknowledged for they confused us frequently, often calling us by each other's name. This was odd, considering how different we are: in style and looks, biographies, and many of our approaches to life. Eve's were intriguingly unique.

"You let your soul go too deep into your body," she reflected at one session. "We have to take up our crosses when we come to earth. We must know when to lay them down to have our hands free for other things." I told her I often bled menstrually when clients brought painful material which naturally touched my own wounds.

"Yes," she responded, "You've gone the inner path. We have to travel it to become honest about ourselves. Now we need to free you up again. For the spirit," she added cryptically.

I painted yellow. I painted blue. I tried to balance them. There was always too much darkness. I could not resist it. My blue crouched heavily at the bottom of the page. The yellow fluttered helplessly above it. When I tried to make them meet a sludgy green appeared – now pale and watery, now dense and inert.

"Think of Scottish hills," said Eve. "Springy turf – green you can walk upon. Not water, not concrete – good solid earth."

I tackle my watery green again. The green concrete seems beyond repair. Eve tells me the story of some early Christian martyr who actually nailed himself to a cross for eight years, then decided he might have made a terrible mistake and unfastened himself again. Poor guy! Let that be a lesson to us all. I feel it does have something to do with me and this business of balancing light and dark. I struggle on. I wish I could begin all over again now I know I must make my yellow more forceful, but this is not to be.

Week after week I stand before the same painting – if, indeed, I could call it that. It's the process, not the product that counts. There are no Michelangelos. I bring red – a few pinkish strokes in the middle of the page. I am terrified. I'll spoil it all.

"More," says Eve. "Now your Ego must arrive." My what? Have I got such a thing? And do I want to declare myself? Eve puts the pressure on. Stroke by stroke the center builds.

"Till it is strong enough to move out." Cautiously I apply another stroke or two.

Eve takes my brush and dashes a great vermilion streak. I yelp. The delicate fabric is ruptured by this bloody gash.

"Stand back now," she commands. I do. Suddenly I feel a surge of excitement. I feel bold. My face grows hot.

"Good," says Eve, watching me. "Now it comes. Off you go."

Under her vigilant care, I step out. Red, loosed from the center, dances towards the periphery – now up, now down, now left, now right. Each stroke requires another somewhere else to balance it. Everything is forgotten in this watchfulness – where next, where does *red* want and need to go? At the end of the hour I am exhausted.

"Lie down," says Eve, fetching woolly rugs. "You must always sense when it is enough. Sometimes a couple of strokes are all you have to do." I am breathing like a runner after a long race. I've been someplace too, though I don't know where. Returning, I also feel revitalized from some secret source.

All through that first winter I paint, sometimes with only one color – yellow upon yellow – till it glows, shines, dances, becomes alive. At home I dare not. Eve suggests I stir the colors in little pots.

"We have to feed the soul. Not just dissect it."

I place three dishes on my kitchen window sill, filled with golden yellow, vermilion, cobalt blue. In between cooking – careful not to mix in these soul ingredients with my meat and potatoes – I swill each round with a little brush according to my mood. Within minutes I feel full of color, no longer shrivelled and grey. I can tackle Michigan winter, even life itself again. My menstrual bleeding lessens each month.

Now I come to red and green again. Though I am afraid, the fear is proper. "A man's destiny begins at the point where his fear lies," declared Carl Jung. This is a threshold crossing into unfamiliar realms and, however often we repeat an exercise, it is always as if we did it for the first time. But I am also more confident now, able to run a few risks.

Each stroke changes the whole, each step takes us somewhere else. What I call "mistakes" – and they look pretty glaring to me – Eve describes as a "new situation". It is one I have given myself to work with, to make something of again. I've told myself – and others – this kind of thing for years. But I've always secretly hoped one could reach the place where one didn't make false moves, could slip through life impeccably. "Sin" means "missing the mark", and I fondly imagined, given a few more years, I might score bulls' eyes every time!

Color instructs me in reality. First I see myself mirrored on the page. Then I try to surrender myself so I can see the color, its nature, its desires. When I follow these, the balance is restored. First on the page, then in me. In each session there may be thirty seconds or so when something astonishing occurs. The colors appear to be alive. I swear I almost see them move without my guiding hand. It is like noticing my child's breathing, the flutter of lashes, when he is dead asleep.

As he wakes, stretches, do I watch, wondering, or lean down and take him in my arms? So with the colors which both need me to sustain their life, yet need to grow free of me. Those moments when I even wonder if they might dance off the page, or I might discover the room and I myself were really made of color all the time, are worth all the hours of struggling with blobs and brushes, ungainly smears, green concrete and the like.

After each session too, I breathe more deeply and easily. My shoulders are relaxed, my feet more firmly planted on the ground. My "hypertrophied" astral body is clearly less strung out. There's a good overall sense of elasticity. What the Rebounder does for my body, color – and Eve – are doing for my soul!

Chapter 11

ORGAN RUBS

"Rub-a-dub dub,
Three men in a tub . . ."
– English Nursery Rhyme.

There is one other significant therapy during this first year – my weekly organ rubs with Dorothea. There is a huge difference, in my experience, between doing something for yourself and having something done for you by another person. I even question the exclusive self-reliance of many healing methods which may deprive us of the gifts that others bring; the intangible yet potent substance that weaves between us to engender healing – stronger perhaps than any medication, any technique.

I recall my first encounter with anthroposophical remedies when I was thrown from a horse and a ring I was wearing bit deep into one finger, nearly to the bone. I neglected the wound. It turned septic. My landlady Joy, a farmer's wife and mother of seven children, noticed it one day and took me immediately to her living room. She made me sit down.

"Calendula," she said with authority, and went to fetch whatever calendula was. She returned with a jar of creamy ointment. I held out my hand for it.

"No." she said. "I must put it on." With great tenderness she smeared my finger. I thanked her and began to get up.

"No, Sit still. I must bandage it." This she did and then sat down herself. Children wailed offstage. She ignored them.

"How are you feeling?"

"Fine. Shouldn't you . . .?" I gestured towards the wails.

"Wait a bit. This should work quite soon." We sat together. Within minutes I felt the inflammation subside. Joy told me calendula was a type of marigold, particularly good for open wounds and fighting infection. As my finger simmered down, I too felt invaded by a rare sense of peace.

"Thank you," I said again, meaning something more this time. Joy smiled.

"It isn't just medicines that heal," she commented. "One must never forget that. Sometimes, if we treat ourselves, they don't even work."

Certainly Dorothea exerted a similar influence. Her three youngest children often shrieked offstage, but she never deflected her consciousness. I was the one who had to bring my focus back to the room, the encounter between my flesh and her fingertips. We meet very intimately through the sense of touch which also, paradoxically, rays us back to ourselves. Besides feeling the quality of Dorothea's presence, I also began to journey into my interior world. The soul has been described as "that savage and beautiful country". The body is no less so; a world of organ, intestine, blood, muscle, lymph, where destruction, metamorphosis and regeneration take place for the most part way below the threshold of consciousness. I can't say I went too far in it, but here and there I would get little intimations of these processes. These evoked a deep awe and reverence for the workings within my own flesh. I felt I had used the resources of my body as if they were inexhaustible capital – as we also deplete the resources of the natural world. The result was breakdown, disease. If I learned nothing more than this in these sessions, it would justify them – a timely reminder of a faulty value system that is bringing humanity to the brink of disaster. Perhaps this illness would educate me in a more responsible participation in world ecology, through attending to the ecology of my own flesh?

The particular massage that Dorothea does is in certain respects different from many methods used today. It is known as Rhythmical Massage and is also part of the anthroposophical package of therapies. Most forms of massage work through directly dissolving the knots and tensions that are lodged in the physical body. Rolfing is a striking example of this. A Rolfer exerts powerful pressure on the afflicted area, which is generally extremely painful. One rhythmical masseur I knew commented that most methods work with the forces of gravity, pressing downward into the physical body. They can be effective and by no means always painful. Rhythmical massage, however works with the forces of levity – aiming to re-enliven the etheric body so that it does the work of healing. (It is the etheric that lifts us out of gravity, as a plant is lifted upward from the earth.)

Thus, like so much of anthroposophical therapy, the problem area is not necessarily tackled directly. If, for example, one suffers from headaches, the usual approach is to massage the shoulders, neck and head. A rhythmical massage would focus on the calves of the legs. In most headaches, the situation is that forces that properly belong in the stomach – metabolic forces, warm and continually active – have trespassed into a region where all should be cool and still. If the calves are massaged, these forces "become interested in what's happening in the lower pole" and return to have a look at what's going on.

I was not allowed a full body massage at this stage. The cancer patient should wait at least six months after surgery lest the mobilized etheric seed the whole body with any stray cancer cells. Dorothea could, however, massage certain organs to stimulate their activity, revitalizing them specifically, and the immune-system generally. These were the "organ rubs."

The first of these was called the sternum rub. What Dorothea actually massaged was the thymus gland. This gland is fist-sized in a child and shrinks to the size of a walnut in the adult or even completely disappears. (This says something about the vitality of childhood, and the degeneration that follows fast on its heels!) Even though the physical organ may have vanished, the "etheric organ" remains. The concept of an invisible etheric organ may be rather hard to grasp, but all our physical organs have their etheric counterparts and treatment is often directed at the latter reality. In the case of an etheric organ whose physical counterpart no longer exists, the notion may seem even more far-fetched! Perhaps the experience many people have after a limb has been amputated and they still feel its presence years afterwards is a good example of this invisible reality.

Dorothea used Silica oil for the sternum (thymus) rub. It was less a "rub" than a rhythmic, snakelike movement down the length of my chest, sometimes in small circles like an interwoven chain, increasing in pressure, then lightening up again. After this rub I found myself breathing deeply, into and out of regions I did not believe my lungs inhabited. I felt expanded, filled with oxygen, able to dispel long pent up poisons, emotions: the general interior clutter reminiscent of my closets and "glory-holes" – those areas in my home upon which I firmly close the doors and hope will never be discovered even by intimate friends!

I recalled a theater director once explaining that the Greeks used drama therapeutically; that people came each year to experience the deep inbreath of terror: "Oooooh-!" followed by the outbreath of relief: "Aaaaah-" This stabilized their breathing rhythms for another year until the plays came round again. This rub seemed to evoke a similar condition. Perhaps it was a modern alternative, given it is not that easy to find a production of Aeschylus any time we realize we have forgotten how to breathe! I thought often of the Greeks, their treasure house of ancient healing wisdom, as I lay in Dorothea's little room, looking out on today's landscape of concrete, steel and plastic, and felt renewed by her competent, tender touch. I told her about my sense of breathing freely again.

"I was taught that if you gave this rub correctly, the patient should breathe differently. If there was no change you knew you hadn't done a good job."

The following week she "rubbed" my liver and spleen. The experience was equally, if more subtly, rewarding. I discovered where my liver is situated, having always vaguely imagined it somewhere in the small of my back! No, it is tidily tucked around my waist as one might carry a small child. My spleen is tucked on the other side. Dorothea told me the spleen must never be massaged on its own; it needs company. It is the organ that mediates between conscious and unconscious realms. I do not now how it does this, but I took her word for it. It can be helped in this function by massage, diet and, I am sure, by working psychotherapeutically. I had no dreams for days after this "rub". I wondered if that were replacing the necessary connection between these realms that dreams make for us.

Dorothea massaged my liver with a figure-eight movement, my spleen in expanding and contracting spirals. She used a different oil for each. Copper for the liver, I remember. Each organ has a specific relation to a certain metal, which in turn connects it to a planet. Though I asked her many questions and strove to remember her answers, I generally sank into such a comfortable semi-conscious state that I forgot them soon afterwards. When she had finished, she would tuck me up under a warm blanket and leave me to rest. I don't know how it is possible to feel energized and relaxed simultaneously, but I did. It was rather like sitting in the bottom of a pot of honey, having eaten half of it. After twenty minutes or so, I would get up and join Dorothea for a cup of wild blackberry tea. We would sit, having interesting conversations about our lives, the lives of others, our hopes for the future, interspersed with equally absorbing exchanges with Sarah, Kirsti and Lauren. Kirsti's main topic was how much of my personal property she could grab from me. She would break into gusty yells whenever I attempted to retrieve my comb or keys. Sarah was often engrossed in being some large unguessable animal; growling and prowling under the table, her intense face hidden behind a curtain of flaming marigold hair. She would emerge to depict these creatures beautifully in crayons and paint.

"That's a bush for the worms to hide in of course," she would tell me sternly. "Or the birds will get them."

"And those?" I ask, pointing at some happy floating pink shapes.

"Flimingos!"

"And these?" Towards big blue shapes hugging the top of the page.

"Oliphants, of course!" Despite my idiocy, Sarah gives me a picture, which I treasure to this day. It is "Mountain Goats. For Lee from dear Sarah". Does anyone dare assert it is my rejuvenated thymus alone that is healing me?

One day Dorothea says: "Irene called. She was really worried about you. She wanted to ask me first how you were doing."

"What did you tell her?"

"I said you were fine. You were doing very well." Dorothea told me that a friend of Irene's whom I slightly know had had some kind of vision that I was very sick and had been trying to contact me to tell me about it. (Thank God he didn't succeed!) Then he had called Irene to off-load on her. Now she was in a state.

"Good God. What do you think is going on?"

"Well, I think basically that cancer scares a lot of people, and they may start imagining all kinds of things that have nothing to do with reality."

"So did you manage to calm everyone down?"

"Yes," said Dorothea with a chuckle. "I told Irene not to forget that life is *the* terminal illness. And we've all got that one!"

Oh, I do like that! Yes – none of us are getting out of this one alive! So hadn't we better make the most of the time we have? I'm certainly enjoying life today, sitting here with Dorothea, Kirsti in my lap, drinking my blackberry tea. Gosh – if I hadn't got cancer I'd be someplace else, unrubbed, untended, and it might not be half as nice as here!

Chapter 12

SPIRITUAL HEALING

*"In my name shall they cast out devils; they shall speak with new
tongues; they shall take up serpents; and if they drink any
deadly thing it shall not hurt them; they shall lay hands on the
sick, and they shall recover. "*
— St. Mark 16:17-18.

There aren't too many people fooling about with serpents or drinking poison
that I know, but there are thousands of spiritual healers and once one is sick one
is bound to run into some, either in literature or in the flesh.

Of course healing is a traditional element in the Christian Church (despite the
founder of Christian Science – Mrs. Eddy – claiming that she had come to restore
it). Every religion has healing rituals, however bizarre some of these may appear
to western "scientific" man. When people say: "I don't believe it," what they are
really saying is: "I want no part of it". It is ridiculous not to believe in something
that clearly exists. It is perfectly reasonable to reject it for oneself. Indeed, it may
prove quite ineffective without one's participating faith. "Thy faith hath made
thee whole," says Jesus on many occasions. Healing undoubtably occurs in the
alchemy between the healer and patient that allows the spirit to enter.

I began to wonder where I stood on this issue and found, as usual, that I had
mixed emotions and views. I believed completely in non-physical healing. I had
the deepest respect for many I had heard of who did it, and those who had
benefited from it. I was very uncertain if I wanted anyone to practise it on me.
Long distance prayers were welcome – very fine, in fact. Imagining an actual
"laying on of hands" made me nervous. This was pretty silly considering I had
once been a patient of a Black Box (Radionics) specialist, sending three or four
of my hairs, no explanation of my symptoms, and was diagnosed and treated
successfully across the Atlantic, sometimes in such uncanny ways that to have a
person in the room, be able to look them in the eye, notice the holes in their socks
or whatever, would surely be less threatening. Anyway, I put that question on the
back burner for a few months.

One young man offered to heal me. I never completely grasped what he said
he did; something to do with taking me out of my body so that I could think pure
thoughts, and then bringing me back in again. These thoughts would then work
into my flesh with positively transforming effects. I could not challenge his

reasoning. Thoughts have a profound effect on our physiology. Norman Vincent Peale, and others, have marketed this insight pretty successfully. A speaker I once heard quoted Charles Darwin as mourning his knowledge that thinking the thoughts he had about evolution had killed his capacity to enjoy music and art toward the end of this life. But I was highly dubious. I did not know if I wanted to leave my body in the hands of this young man while I scooted off someplace else. I wound up refusing his offer, grateful that he had made it, and we parted friends.

My mother wrote about a well known healer in Norfolk, England, called Matthew Manning. He was treating large numbers of people successfully. He had a particular gift with children, apparently. He had actually destroyed cancer cells in a test tube, by spiritual means, under the gaze of several members of the medical profession. He was booked months in advance. Could she make an appointment for me this summer? She sent me several of his tapes. I listened to these. I enjoyed his pleasant, unassuming English voice. He sounded down-to-earth, modest, compassionate. I was not too keen on the visualizations he included, backed by some pretty dramatic sound effects. Full blown cavalry charges with trumpets and pounding hooves accompanied the attack of white blood cells. Something between a monsoon and a burst pipe represented the malignant cells being washed away. But that was my problem with visualization, obviously now compounded by an auditory complex too. Even allowing for that, I couldn't get round to making a date.

One question I had was: "Do I actually want someone else to do the job for me?" That isn't quite the right way of putting it. A quite active surrender to the process of healing, and to a greater power, would be asked of me and that could be as difficult as anything. I daren't even jump off the edge of a swimming pool. How much more would I need to let go with a spiritual healer? It might well be the great lesson of this disease. I suspected I might be resisting for quite the wrong reason.

Yet, there was still something in that question for me. Partly, I did not feel ready to be told that the threat to my life had been completely removed before I had made the changes I knew this illness called for. I needed the reminder, the provocation to my awareness, without which I could all too easily fall back into old ways. I had not, in fact, left any of these old ways, to my frustration and shame. But for all my stuckness, I did long for some kind of transformation and if that occurred without my conscious participation, I knew I would be at some level profoundly dissatisfied.

In all these musings, I think I had a rather muddled association between spiritual healing and the prevalent contemporary fashion in America for being "Born Again". I certainly do not wish to decry moments of spiritual rebirth – or indeed any opportunity to make a fresh start. But much of what I see happening in this country in various movements for religious renewal troubles me deeply. (The Master Race consciousness – the Saved and Damned – that afflicts some groups is, of course, quite terrifying, but that was not the issue here.) My concern is that being "reborn" too often licenses a rejection of the past and any responsibilities we may still have to the consequences of actions performed in it. Americans seem to have a peculiar ability to obliterate the past – perhaps stemming from the pioneering spirit that sought a New Land and a New Life. While admirable in many ways, it has a shadow side. And I do not believe we can find a true future without a remembered past. "Without memories," says Dame Eyola, in *The Never-Ending Story*, "it is impossible to wish." I think, in submitting to a spiritual healing, I worried that I might be deprived of some vital part of my history. I think I was wrong about this. But something was holding me back.

Then I met Nan. My friend Joyce, an American and fellow student in our counseling training many years ago, wrote from England sending me Nan's address. This had been given her by a mutual friend of theirs, a Jungian analyst living in Connecticut. Nan was a healer living in Detroit. Quite a round-about contact, then, and one which reflected Joyce's concern in a way that moved me deeply. Joyce is a fine, discriminating person whose recommendations can always be taken on trust. So I did decide to contact Nan. Before I could, I got a card from her. She mentioned nothing about spiritual healing, only that she hoped we might meet, having friends in common and probably a lot else besides. I called her up. We set a lunch date at the Traffic Jam & Snug.
"How will we recognize each other?" I asked.
"Oh, I'll know you," said Nan. If she hadn't sounded so down-to-earth, and delightfully warm, I should have been alarmed. Did her powers extend to recognizing a stranger in a crowded restaurant? And what else might be visible, if this were the case? I'd need to fluff up my aura, as well as remember to wear clean underwear!

We actually recognized each other easily. We spent a few hours together in rare conversation, touching on themes I seldom speak of, being too close to the heart. That they were close to hers opened a space for them, and surrounded our words with tranquil silences.

She told me she was a recent convert to Catholicism – a "dissenting convert" – drawn mainly by the power of the Eucharist. (I didn't tell her then, but I may one day, that my first request of God on learning I had cancer was that I might "see" spiritually the transubstantiation before I died.) I am strongly drawn to dissenting Catholics, respecting their commitment to the spirit that so often works in strange and wonderful ways through the frequently outworn forms of the Catholic Church.

By coffee, Nan had said nothing about healing, and I thought it time to ask her what she actually did. She said she honestly did not know and her concern with what might be working through her when she healed was one driving power towards formal religion again. As Edgar Cayce had struggled so movingly with the question of the origin of his own powers and the morality of exercising them without his full consciousness, so had Nan questioned how she might protect herself and others if she were to use this gift. She had discovered it through healing warts on her son's hands while praying for him at bedtime. And, despite the skepticism of her husband, a medical doctor, she had continued to effect other cures. I was quite fascinated by her factual, modest story, and deeply impressed by her moral integrity. As we paid our bills, I found myself asking:

"What would you think about doing a healing on me?" Nan looked surprised. I don't think it had occurred to her, though I'd explained about my cancer earlier. "I mean, I thought that's what Joyce had in mind, when she introduced us – though I'm awfully glad we met anyway."

"Oh, so am I," responded Nan warmly. "I hope we'll see more of each other."

"Me too. Let's keep in touch. And would you think about a healing? And I'll think about it too. I mean, we could both sleep on the idea?" Despite the ease between us, I suddenly feel quite embarrassed at asking her – is it an imposition? Am I really ready for this?

Nan gives me a deep look, then chuckles as she buttons up her coat. "You look terribly well, you know," she says. "Well, let's see how it goes."

*   *   *

Nan and I haven't had that formal healing session yet. A year later Sister Marcia, a Catholic nun, performed a healing on me. Through her laying on of hands, prayers and, I think, some speaking in tongues, a new mass in my breast disappeared the following night. A difficult relationship was also healed. My false opinions were corrected, happily. In the intervening time, however, I often thought of Nan, and I believe our conversation together was a spiritual healing of a kind.

Chapter 13

PROGRESS?

*"When medicine just consists of treatment to physical symptoms
it makes sense to talk of it in terms of success and failure. But
when we set out to heal ourselves . . . we embark on a journey
. . . for its own sake, not to reach a specific destination. All
travellers always arrive eventually."*
> – The Bristol Programme, Penny Brohn.

Within a few months I expected result. I demanded them. I was giving 80%
of my time, money and energy to licking this disease. What was there to show
for it other than a diminishing bank account? I wanted someone to show up
bearing a red rosette and silver trophy, rather as I used to fantasize the outcome
of childhood hunter trials, even while knowing I would probably flunk the first
fence. "Bravo! Well ridden!" I could canter round the arena triumphantly. No
more cancer. Not a single cell. And never again to come unto me!

Wanting incontrovertible proof was also tied up with what I fondly thought
of as "the rest of my life"; the diminished area that was not concerned with cancer
and that contained such things as work, love, play, my purpose etc. I guess I was
stuck with the notion that Life After Cancer could be much like Life B.C. I could
pick up the threads again with maybe a few extra colorful ones now woven in. I
did not seem able to grasp the fact that having cancer was now so firmly woven
into it that all the patterns might have changed.

I worried about barely working quite a lot. Though my parents had offered
to back me up financially through this illness, I felt a new thrust to my work life
might signal triumph over the disease. I confess I imagined an onrush of clients
who all had cancer too! I, from the depths of my wisdom and experience, would
gently guide them through their crises. Their fees would underwrite my
expensive therapies. I extended this vision to include a Cancer Center modelled
somewhat on the Bristol Programme; Lenny, Dorothea, Eve and myself as chief
protagonists. Eve had also had cancer diagnosed and treated a couple of months
after me. Together we had formidable resources; tons of literature and tons of
different experiences. While I bounced on my trampoline, Eve gulped wheat-
grass juice. She attended Reach for Recovery programs. I experimented with
images of sharks. A doctor, a nurse and masseure, an art therapist and a counselor
– we made an impressive team. I imagined our clinic down to the vegetarian
lunches, the color of the walls.

I was way off beam. Certainly no-one had the remotest interest to turn to me because they were a cancer patient. Those who trickled in by early spring had any problem but that one. The headings of love, play, my purpose offered as little evidence of success. Surely God didn't only intend that I become a champion juicer of carrots? He must have something more in mind for me than perfecting this minor science?

I looked to my body next. There is really no way of knowing that you haven't got a single cancer cell. I did see that. I owned reluctantly that it would take years without a recurrence to confirm bodily health. But I searched for subtle signs that I might have turned the tide; that the process of the past twenty years, peaking in cancer, might now be on the ebb. Others noticed radical changes in a short time. Beata Bishop, following the Gerson regime, lost her arthritis and diabetes within two weeks. Within a year or so her grey eyebrows had grown back brown! Dr. Anthony Sattilaro, on the macrobiotic diet, saw surplus weight, puffy eyes, sallow skin, vanish abruptly. Everyone recorded increased vitality, creativity, profound psychological changes almost overnight. Not so myself!

I needed at least ten hours of sleep each night; rather more than previously. I still had dark circles under my eyes. There were definitely a few more grey streaks in my hair. I might be about to beat the world record for keeping the sediment lining my intestines intact. Cheri had estimated that 8-10 weeks of colonics would begin to shift the deeper layers. She told me I would know when that happened. I noticed nothing, and she confirmed that nothing had.

I knew my regime of therapies and diet was not 100% pure. I still had my organic coffee. I was not entirely sugar free. But could these minor defections really hold me back? I still consumed a lot of nervous energy simply accomplishing the daily round; shopping, getting the car fixed, changing light bulbs, making lunchboxes, as well as fitting in my therapies. I could not see how to slow things down. I reflected wryly that the angels, or whoever sends us forth to accomplish our destinies, obviously fail to reckon with blocked plumbing or flat car batteries! If I did slow down and give my astral body a bigger break, our lives would surely grind to a halt. I felt resentful. I felt depressed. There was no time for work anyway, and there might never be again.

One marginal improvement I noticed was that I had got better at saying NO. I refused to bake cakes for Adam's school fairs – quite possibly to everyone's vast relief, since my cakes leave a lot to be desired! Nor did I attend the innumerable meetings with which our community abounds. I still linked my refusals to the fact that I had cancer, that I'd recently undergone surgery. People were shocked and sympathetic. How would they feel three years from now? I used the disease to extricate myself from burdensome commitments. Some books make a great deal of this: Why do you need your illness, etc.? Learning to say "No" is considered by many to be a prime lesson of this particular disease. Perhaps the day would come when I would merely say "No - I don't want to," without adding cancer as the excuse? Might I end up not wanting to do anything at all?

This led to the awesome question: Do I want to get well? If the only obvious change was a gradual vanishing from the earthly scene, perhaps this was the case? This thought frightened me a lot. I tiptoed around the brink of it for a long time. "Why are you still drinking coffee, when you know it's bad for you?" "Because I like the taste." As I lowered myself gently into this one, icy feelings swirled about me, dark currents tugged me into depths I seldom dive to if I can avoid it. Yes, indeed, there is a part of me that would love to give up, that resists life – its joys and sorrows, its responsibilities. It is this part that stages such delightful memorial services for myself; where people celebrate my virtues, mourn the deep loss to the human community. Was I secretly gripped by Thanatos? Was this the reason I was making no progress that I could see?

Around this time I go for my next check-up mammogram. It is about as painful as anything can be. I have only three-quarters of my very small breast to load on to the machine. What remains is filled with large red sore lumps; a final glorious reaction to the *Iscador*. I nearly pass out, and have only the warmth and sensitivity of the radiologist to thank for preventing me. The nurse also discovers new tender knobby patches in my right breast and prescribes an X-ray for that one too. "Oh God, not this one now!" I am shaking with anxiety.

When the doctor comes into the cubicle where I am waiting shivering in my cotton gown, she greets me cheerfully, places her hand firmly on top of my closed file and enquires:

"And how old is your son?"

"Nine." Lord, not that one! She is really going straight for the jugular. How is it that someone I like and respect, and appears to care for me, can turn the blade deep in my most vulnerable place? I can't even protest. I have no defence, as I might against someone else.

"I thought you'd said 'nine'," she comments vaguely. Her hand is still ominously on my file. I can't look her in the eyes. I know what I'll see. She's obviously found another malignancy. I begin to shake inwardly.

"Tell me," she says, while I try to gather myself into a more coherent shape. "What are you going to do if you have a recurrence?"

"I don't know," I say wildly. "I'll have to think about it."

"No. I want to know now."

"What would my options be?"

"Well, we couldn't do another lumpectomy. It would have to be a full mastectomy this time. Plus further treatment of course."

"I am in treatment," I babble. "Haven't you seen my mistletoe lumps? I'm doing masses of treatments." She gives me another look. I can feel it, but I'm still not going to look at her.

"I mean radiation. Why have you refused radiation?" She doesn't even ask accusingly. Just "Why", why would I do such a thing? This is worse than disobeying a favorite teacher; worse than the time I cut all the flowers in my mother's garden and then, full of four-year old remorse, tried desperately to stick them on their stalks again. And I don't have a good answer now. Everything that led to my rejection of this treatment goes into a big blur. I forget Pamela Benitez calling me in excitement to report those experts who could not decide if it had a value or not. I forget Dr. Fried recommending I concentrate on *Iscador*. Above all, I forget my own soul-searchings, my own questions. Pretty silly, some of these more abstruse ponderings, particularly when I cannot know the answers now, or perhaps ever. At the time they seemed important. Now they appear ridiculous – just another instance of my general idiocy. I'm in a flat panic now. I hear our conversation continuing as if other people were conducting it.

I say something about conventional treatments simply buying time. They are not cures. The doctor disagrees.

"In your case I think we could call it a cure. Radiation offers a 98% chance of there being no recurrence within five years, 95%-93% of none in ten." Over this hang the words she has the charity not to repeat:

"What about your son?"

"And without radiation?" I enquire, with somewhat precarious poise.

"I expect a recurrence within two years."

"Have I got one now?" It can hardly be worse, and her hand is still glued to my wretched file.

"No. Not this time." Well, there's one good breath drawn since we started this interview.

She mentions the doctor I saw at the ROC. My mind is still so fuzzy, I am not sure why she brought her up. Perhaps she thinks I might change my mind and have radiation at this point?

"She said if I didn't come right away, she wouldn't treat me." The doctor smiles knowingly. She'd soon sort that one out.

"Besides, I don't think I could work with her."

"Well, we can easily find you someone else." She mentions casually that my tumors, none larger than 0.3cm, had each contained approximately four million cells and only one needed to escape to start the whole thing up again. I respond with a little more vigor than I feel:

"I am having treatment you know. Lots of treatment actually. *Iscador*, diet, healing movement, exercise. . ."

"I know that," she replies briskly. "I'm talking about treatment we know works." I try a last desperate bid:

"Why is it Dr. Martino is so supportive then? Why will she have me as a patient, if I'm a lost cause?"

"Well, you mustn't forget that you do offer us the opportunity to observe the process of this disease. That's always interesting."

I think she said "process" not "progress", or is it the same thing? I'm beyond the finer details at this point. I'm off into a vivid fantasy of myself as doomed guinea pig of the orthodox community; Dr. Martino relishing my inevitable demise – an interesting piece of research, another nail in the coffin of alternative medicine, (foolhardy enough to challenge the High Priests of Science,) as my own coffin is prepared for me. Have I made a ghastly mistake? In my pride and stupidity have I also chosen wholly and solely for myself? Disregarded Adam and his needs, my responsibilities? Such thoughts are unbearable, and I sense I'd better get out of here quick so that I can confront them in the comfort and privacy of my own home.

"And what if I'm still alive and kicking a few years from now?" I ask, with a papery grin, gathering my robe about me with as much dignity as I can muster. "I'll buy you lunch," says the doctor, adding firmly: "And I sincerely hope you are."

As we part, she extracts one commitment from me.

"Will you promise to have a mammogram every six months."

"Yes, I'll do that."

"Promise me now."

"OK. I promise."

Driving home on the freeway, feeling battered way beyond my aching breast the muddle begins to clear. I don't mean it gets any easier. The truths that now loom up through my foggy consciousness are the great bitter truths we may take a lifetime, maybe longer, to learn. One is, of course, that we can't please everyone. Even those we respect and like – as I actually do this doctor – may stand on opposing ground. Another is that there is no "right" or "wrong" way to go. There is simply what each of us elects to do. Life is not a multiple-choice exam, with the correct answer waiting to be recognized. And sadly, we are not educated to trust our own powers of discernment, to risk our unique, existential responses to our individual destinies. We still hope and long for the simplicity and certainty of there being a good or bad thing to do. The truth is, however, that each choice we make brings certain consequences and requires a sacrifice of other directions, other possibilities. Walking one path leaves others untrodden, and we cannot retrace our steps. We head off, too, into the darkness, only later able to see where this path has led us. And we cannot know beforehand – (that is the lure and delusion of causal thinking, programs, statistics, for these exclude the future, the unknown, unborn potentials, the "never befores" in ourselves and the life of the world.)

What I am facing now, somewhere along the Chrysler Freeway, is, quite simply the choice I have made – for better or worse – and the fact that I have to stand in it. It will bring an ongoing tension between myself and some members of the conventional medical community, unless I choose to walk away from them. And I do not intend to do that. So I must learn to trust my own resources, while respecting theirs – for this is my illness, my life, my death. And ultimately, whatever happens I can praise or blame no-one but myself. This realization touches infantile longings to make others responsible: "My Mum made me wear these horrible gloves!" How often have I resorted to this kind of evasion of personal responsibility, and how much more terrifying is this particular issue – a whole lot bigger than whether I get a new haircut, or sell my car, or take a vacation in New Mexico! For heaven's sake, this is a matter of life or death!

I pull into my driveway. A new thought hits me like a rock. "You don't want to die." What? What was that? "Don't you think what you've just gone through tells you you want to live?" Wow! I suppose it does. Get thee behind me, Thanatos, I'm off to other things!

A while later Cynthia says: "I don't want to state the obvious. But since you're looking for signs of progress, don't you think not having a recurrence yet is pretty good?" Lord Almighty, it's staring me straight in the face. I think my biggest problem is not cancer, but thinking straight.
"You'll have to state the obvious," I tell her. "Till I get it into my thick head."

These episodes, however, are still not enough. I want positive evidence, not just an X-ray negative. I try to slow down, do things more rhythmically, step up my meditation times. Once in a while I discover I am enjoying the pace for its own sake. Adam and I do not fall off the edge of the world, either, when I mop my kitchen floor phlegmatically, or exchange ten minutes of fretfully complaining that I don't have enough time to actually use this time constructively. I do my daily eurythmy faithfully, trusting that it is doing something to restore harmony. I notice no changes here, and after some weeks call Alice in Pennsylvania, as agreed, for a progress report.
"How are you doing?"
"I don't know really. I am doing it."
"Good. Do you feel any warmer?"
"Well – no. I don't think so. Mind you, it's pretty cold here right now."
"Yes. Don't worry. It takes time. The eurythmy and the *Iscador* will begin to work together. Maybe in six months you'll notice a difference." Gosh, six months more! How immensely comforting. So is Alice; her warm, calm voice infusing me with hope over all these miles.
"Do it without desire," she tells me. "And let's talk again in another month or so."

Next morning I tackle the movements again. Without desire! I know what she means. Without shopping lists floating in my head; without gazing at my pear tree through the window and wondering when the first buds will open; without even imagining the next movement – simply staying within the one I am doing. Real Zen stuff this. And about as hard as anything I've attempted, caught as I am in a lifelong habit of the five-year plan. Without desire, too, for any particular experience as I actually move each step and gesture. I try and try again.

Suddenly, unbidden and unhoped for, I feel as I lift my arms as if I'm lifting a light cloak too; as if there's this invisible substance surrounding me, that I move within and that moves within me. It is extraordinary. A quite definite yet delicate fabric of currents that, if I move too abruptly I rupture, rather as one's arm might break through water when swimming, yet far subtler. Somewhere between air and water perhaps. Somewhat overcome, I lie down under my wooly rugs. I feel the same delicate movement along my forearms and legs. Is it warmth? Warmth seems too strong a word. But there is something going on.

Next day I wait for it to happen again. Nothing. Alice's words return. "Without desire". I guess I cannot even hope for a repeat. Off I go again, as undesirously as I can. Fail, try, fail, try again. Sometimes for a few seconds I feel it. It is like those brief moments in painting when the colors flicker into life. But these moments are rare and many mornings my body blunders about in a space that feels empty and arid, devoid of such living energies.

Do the rare moments prove anything anyway? I am clearly hard to please and still caught in the success or failure alternatives. I know this is not what healing is about, but I beg for one really good sign and then I'll stop demanding any more.

I choose my eyesight as the litmus test. Three years ago, Lulu and I got reading glasses when we discovered together in a downtown restaurant that we couldn't read the numbers in the telephone book. We had wanted to call Mary-Jo to join us, and that day we had to eat without her. We have reached the same point, with our glasses, again. I actually believe the latest telephone book has been issued in a smaller print. I've noticed they've reduced the print on medicine bottles too this year. Whether or not I am the victim of a conspiracy, I am determined to hold out a few more weeks, though Lulu is ready to capitulate and suggests we go to the same optometrist so we can help each other choose fancy frames. I refuse. I am drinking a few gallons of carrot juice daily and probably eating more Hunza apricots than the Hunzas themselves (who retain perfect vision till aged 140 or so.) It can only be a matter of a few more weeks before all these good things resurrect my optic nerves. I peer at the small print resolutely, awaiting the hour when it miraculously sharpens under my gaze. Lulu goes her way and comes to supper one evening with a bold new pair of spectacles in glossy scarlet frames.

The weeks pass. The struggle to decipher print intensifies, but I still expect to win. It is when I am planning to fly to Chicago that I am finally stumped. I cannot read the street map. I am not even certain what is City and what is Lake. I dare not travel this blind, and hastily repair to the optometrist. I console myself with a more modest version of Lulu's frames; the upper edge an unobtrusive crimson, and return somewhat mollified. I put them on at supper to show Adam. "You look a real dork in those," he comments. (I gather "dork" is a sort of super-jerk in current idiom.)

"How come?" I protest. "How can Lulu have scarlet frames and I look a dork in these? The red hardly shows!"

"You're not Lulu," he replies.

That is incontestable. I am not Lulu. I am not a beautiful woman with wild, curly gold and silver hair. I can't wear one earring, blue and black zebra-striped longjohns, a man's jacket and silver buckled Victorian boots. (I could, but I'd

probably be locked up.) I don't make everyone feel wherever I go as if they've just drunk a couple of glasses of vintage champagne. Beyond the fact that we were born two days apart – she in Windsor, Ontario and I in Windsor, England – we have few resemblances. I am reflecting on this when Adam, who probably noticed how crestfallen I look, makes a supreme effort – Lulu has a very high place in his heart – and says, guardedly:
"Well, Lulu did look a bit dorkish too."

So here I am: a half-blind dork, occasionally able to sense energy currents, under some pressure to expect recurring malignancies within the next eighteen months, crumbling into bed with all my wrinkles and grey hairs at around nine o'clock each night. Perhaps it *is* time to stop begging for trophies and embark upon the journey for its own sake.

Chapter 14

EXPLORER

"You must go too far before you know how far to go."
– Andre Gide.

If this is a journey, have I any idea where I have come from or where I might be going? Blundering about in this new country, I've been mainly preoccupied with the physical aspects of travelling: the next meal, the continual checking of emergency supplies. I may well resemble those tourists who miss the glories of temple, shrine, colorful bazaar, because they don't trust the water, or the natives, or are unwilling to forgo their afternoon tea. What am I missing as I obsessively juice my carrots, wallow in fever baths, ritually imbibe my medicines? Though there have been many novel experiences, lacking some sense of meaning, this expedition may leave me as ignorant and untouched as if I had stayed at home.

Nancy visits one day, bringing me two beautiful, quite different pieces of white coral – one for each hand – and a charming mandala woven of wool and bamboo and feathers that she made at a workshop on the Indian Medicine Wheel. "What dreams have you had?" She asks immediately, for dreams *are* the royal road to the unconscious and, as therapists, one of our own most immediate ways of sharing what is really going on.

"None to speak of," I say. She gives me a very direct look. Then we both chuckle. There are often dreams we would much rather not speak of, but which are extremely important nonetheless!

"Honestly," I tell her. "I've barely remembered any since this thing began. I don't think I'm blocking a lot of vital material. I know I'd feel it somewhere if I was."

"Yes, you would, wouldn't you. Well, it's certainly interesting."

She shares a couple of pretty powerful dreams of her own and I can feel these touching me, triggering deep feelings in response to her, and also towards myself. We both sit on my back porch and have a little weep. A very refreshing and connecting interlude. I remind her that that is often the way between us – her dream evoking my waking experience and vice versa.

"So what about your waking experience then? Have you any sense of what it's all about?" No, I guess I don't. I guess I haven't really begun to ask, explore. The question of when to interpret and when to allow the psyche to inform us in ways beyond words and concepts is important. We both know that. But it's been quite a while to live in a cloud of unknowing, and Nancy's visit makes me wonder if an end to this time might be at hand.

79

"I'm a slow starter," I tell her ruefully, as she gets up to leave. "My birth was induced, you know. I probably need you to apply the psychological forceps once in a while."

My sister, Sukie, is another catalyst.
"How are you working with it?" She asks on one of her long distance calls that I always appreciate. She is adept at working psychologically with physical states. She uncovers mother complexes in ovarian cysts, an early trauma in a sore throat. I admire this greatly and have respectfully watched her emerge into the fine person and healer of others that she is.
"Well, I don't really know," I admit. "Too busy sleeping or drinking carrot juice."
"Do you do visualization?"
"Well, sometimes – when I get round to it." I think, with shame, of my munching, winking sharks. I even forgot my bouncing, sappy episodes this week.

We talk some more. She recounts a little of her own most recent process and the various methods that have led her to still deeper self discoveries. All this is by way of encouragement. I am truly grateful and genuinely perplexed that I seem to be doing so little for myself in this realm. The physical therapies are, in fact, subtly affecting it. Since taking the *Iscador* I feel "lighter" in some indefinable way. Other patients speak of this, so I presume it's the *Iscador*. After painting or massage I'm often pervaded by a lovely sense of peace. My terrors about Adam, our life together, my possible demise, surface less frequently. But what am I doing consciously? Am I simply allowing the remedies to do the work and failing to take over where they leave off?

Since I have no inkling of how I arrived in cancer country or what I'm supposed to be doing now that I'm here, I turn to others who have charted the territory. Most sensible travellers rely on maps and I do have to wonder why I have taken so long to spread some out.

Physical medicine is, naturally, concerned with the physical terrain. Dr. Martino, interested in a build-up of body fats as a possible cause, did my chloresterol count. It was under half the national average, so it didn't appear to be that. There are other tentative hypotheses as to how we might have landed here – genetic and/or environmental factors seem to be the chief routes. Important information, no doubt, but about as satisfying as a list of airline and train times would be in a travelog. Its chief function is – again by physical means – to effect our escape as quickly as possible. What one might find in this country, or even bring back from our sojourn, is not its concern. And while it's a comfort to know there are people around with ropes and machetes, they are not the ones to teach us about the history and culture of this land.

When we move into the psychological realm, there are only too many waiting to enlighten us. Despite the ascending piles of books and pamphlets – many of which I have spent my own good money on – I have remained an obstinately poor student of whatever wisdom they contain. Impelled by Nancy and Sukie, perhaps now by some part of myself, I tackle the literature again. It doesn't take long before I'm thoroughly depressed.

It appears there is something so deeply and gravely wrong with every cancer patient that the cancer itself is really the least of our worries. Our souls, our personalities, are in such bad shape, we should hardly mind our bodies sprouting a few lumps and bumps. Though I feel myself bristling with distaste and shame, I read on in the hope of finding a more heartening account. No such luck. Though couched in a tone of encouragement and hope, and offering myriad ways of effecting radical change, what we have to change is a pretty dismal mess. What begins to congeal from the numerous theories on offer is The Cancer Personality. This is variously described as: helpless, cold, withdrawn, victimized, full of bitterness and despair, unable to laugh, love, rage, weep enough, (what is enough?) unable to say "No", unable to endure stress, unable to do anything much except buckle under and get cancer. Furthermore, we present a benign exterior – the sickening saccharine do-gooders of the world – while festering malignantly within. We have poor self-images and low self-esteem, (small wonder, if that's the way we are!) We long ago lost our creativity – if we ever had any in the first place. Getting cancer is a last desperate bid for change, an attempt to get attention from others and, hopefully, from ourselves. Then – I suppose – we can rage, weep, laugh, love etc., as never before and this will heal us, whatever it does for those around us. They will have to take care of themselves for a change.

Of course I can find myself mirrored in these descriptions. I once bit a bedspread till four of my teeth fell out. How long is it since I expressed such violent passion? The tears I've held back would fertilize the Sahara with dozens of green oases. I cannot count the times I've said "Yes" when I really meant "No". I've created nothing in this life that I can see, since I proudly brought home some grubby little woven mats from school. Why then do I find myself resisting this picture so strenuously? Is it merely that I've spent so many years shedding my identification with the Capricorn Personality of astrology and am reluctant to take on its even less alluring counterpart? Is it the natural aversion most of us feel when we first uncover the unsavory truth about ourselves? If it fits, surely I have a moral obligation to put it on. Summing up our common state, one pundit writes: "Of all causes in the cancer-process in every shape, neurotic agencies are the most powerful." Well, I certainly am neurotic. And I do have cancer. How can I challenge this judgement, brought by an expert with more fancy letters after his name than I have in my name itself? Lenny had told me I have all the appropriate psychological patterns – a polite way of referring to what are clearly a legion of shadowy complexes. But even while my mind is acknowledging the impeccable logic behind all these statements, and their probable fit with me, somewhere in my diaphragm a fist begins to clench, readying itself to punch a hole in them.

Things reach a climax when, moving up (or down?) the psycho-spiritual ladder, I encounter the blanket theory that we create our own reality. I'd sensed this idea lurked behind much of the psychological material. I had even cast furtive glances at it from time to time, then quickly turned my head away. I'm faced with confronting it head on when someone I vaguely know approaches me in the street one day. He advances cheerily, gives me an encouraging, pitying smile and says: "Sorry to hear you have cancer. But it's all in the mind of course, isn't it?"

"Mine's not," I reply. "Mine's in my body actually." I say this rather too loudly, and feel myself turning pink.

"Well – er, I know that. But what I mean is the mind creates these things, doesn't it? And then you can use your mind to change it all around."

"Who created my mind?" I enquire. I'm still speaking too loudly. My toes are curled inside my sneakers because I can't actually dig them into the sidewalk. But that's what I'm doing metaphorically. It's time to put my foot down, to stand my ground.

"Oh – you know what I'm trying to say . . ."

"You're trying to tell me that I made this happen. That I create my destiny – single-handed – no help or hindrance from anyone, anything . . ."

"Well, not exactly –"

"Yes, that's exactly what you're telling me. And I'm not going to take it. I'm not that omnipotent. And I won't feel that guilty –"

"Hey – don't take it so strong. I never meant . . ."

I'm very red now, and feeling very rude, but I can't stop myself.

"That's just the kind of destructive message I've had enough of. People could die of guilt, not cancer –"

"I only wanted to help. I've got a fantastic book. I'll lend it to you. You can make anything happen. It shows you how . . ."

"Well, not right now thanks . . ." I'm beginning to simmer down into a low boil of shame. It isn't his fault. He does mean well. (I'm struck, however, with the contradiction that I must still purchase expensive books, or cures, from the purveyors of the self-heal notion.)

"Thanks for the offer, though." We both trail into some general niceties to cozy up the encounter, and go our separate ways.

I stomp off down the streets. No, I mutter vehemently, surprising several passers-by. NO, NO, NO. How many people do I know who died of cancer and in no way resemble the Cancer Personality? Quite a few, now I come to think of it. I suspect thousands of wise, creative, integrated beings have succumbed to this disease. How many others do I know who in some way or other fit the type and yet continue in perfect health? Though many cancer patients may indeed own some, even all, of these dismal characteristics, couldn't the same be said for a large percentage of the human race that the clinician and theorist never get to meet?

The notion that we each are sole creator of our own reality infuriates me even more. I know there's a thread of truth that needs teasing out of this blanket, but it's not the whole truth by any manner of means. Of course much of who we are, and have been is manifest in an illness. It does belong to us so to speak. And there is much we can do in becoming at least co-responsible for whatever healing may take place. But there's a vast difference between owning my illness and imagining I caused it. To assume I am sole creator of this, or any other event, seems to me to be an unpardonable arrogance, narcissism and spiritual blindness. How can it possibly be said that I and I alone control and order my destiny? Are those thousands of people living near Chernobyl responsible for their cancer? Did those who build the reactor and failed to maintain it efficiently have no part to play? Our lives are influenced, shaped and guided by so many others, so many factors, that only a four-year old could reason otherwise. And don't we attempt to grow out of such infantile and omnipotent fantasies? This egocentric and isolationist view also deprives us of the rich, complex, wonderful mystery of our interconnectedness, and the hope of our continuing existence within its web. Why would I bother with friendship, starlight, birdsong, by whose grace I am fashioned, if everything that happens is made by me?

NO, NO, NO. I continue prowling the streets because I think better with my feet than with my head. Once I stop and chuckle. How's that for a Cancer Personality? If I've failed to say No enough times in my life, I'm certainly making up for it now. But as I turn for home I see there are still some steps to take. I may know what I am fighting against. Do I know what I'm fighting for? "*Neti, Neti* . . .not this, not that," is a time-honored way of self-discovery. There should come a point where we say: "Yes – this is it." Before I burn all the maps, hadn't I better set out to draw a few of my own?

Chapter 15

QUESTIONS

"Only that which is fruitful is true."
— Goethe.

The trouble with all the theories I've encountered so far is that they only describe one part of the truth. It's like baking a cake with half the ingredients missing; bound to be unappetizing, if not downright inedible. Pondering this, wise words of my English friend and mentor, David, return. "Honour the resistance. It is in the tension between what drives us forward and what holds us back that we find our true direction." I begin to feel this in a deeper way, and questions surface in response.

Are our lives guided as surely and fatefully by our blocks and complexes as by our positive impulses, as the course of a river is shaped by its banks, its torrent dammed or diverted by rock and boulder so that it seeks and finds its own particular pace and course? Without such shaping would we too not leak and seep into undifferentiated swamp? There can be no splendor of eddy, pool or waterfall without the barrier of granite, the sudden crumbling of soft earth. So am I not kept on course, my flow sculpted by just those parts of myself that seem to stand in my way? Have I been led to this point just as purposefully by my weaknesses as by my strengths, and might I need them still to get where I want to go? Imagining this puts my past patterns in quite a new light and softens the sense of guilt and shame.

If this is so, where shall I look now? In concocting my theory, I need to add one vital missing ingredient. This is our sense for the future as well as the past. As creatures embedded in time, this holds the other half of our reality. Ten years down the road this event will look quite different; the picture, extended by further insights, further experiences, will have acquired other tones, shapes, colorings; a wider landscape surrounding the single phenomenon of my cancer which now, like a rock, obtrudes into my vision so that I see nothing beyond. "We walk backwards, in darkness, into our future," once commented one of the wise old men in my life. "We can only see the past extending in front of us. What's coming to meet us is hidden from our gaze." That image stayed with me. I usually sit with my back to the engine on a train journey so I can see the landscape relatively effortlessly. Things tend to loom, rush by too suddenly, facing the other way – as they do in life itself. But I must honor the unknown substance awaiting me if

I am to be true to reality. Without it I am prey to the great illusion of causal thinking that believes we can unlock the secrets of our biographies by turning to the past alone. Do the roots of a plant tell us the shape of its future leaves and blossoms, upon which who knows what winds will blow, what light or water fall? Obviously not. How much less so can we know our own becoming; each human being a species to itself, capable of illimitable diversity.

Perhaps it is the idea of what we might become, and our urge to realize this, that fashions our origins, magnetically draws the events that seek us, (the longing to join the sea that causes the spring to bubble up from the heart of distant hills?) Thus our causes could as well live in the future as in the past. I share this perspective – perhaps not original, but now inspiring me – with Mary-Ellen, my tutor from Marygrove, as we walk back from lunch one day and we agree it is as valid as the other way around.

Together we also challenge the Calvinist (and indeed Catholic!) emphasis on guilt and sin that dominates so many of our current attitudes. Even in our Judaeo-Christian tradition there are more creative ways of looking at the trials that beset us. "Happy the man whom God chastiseth," says Proverbs, and Jesus puts his disciples firmly in their places when they enquire whose sin has caused a man to be born blind. "Not this man's sin, nor his father's sin. This is for the glory of God." How I cherish my dialogues with Mary-Ellen and, talking with her, I feel a shift of inner ground, to a place where I can breathe a freer air. "Your cancer" another friend, and psychic, had said, "is the doorway to your next space." It feels truer to look ahead, or even examine these portals than to turn back.

I must be listening better these days, for another voice now speaks – Fred Duhl's from our training days at the Boston Family Institute. "Not *causes – consequences!*" he declaims. Again and again Fred dragged us, mainly by the power of his own passion, out of the caverns of the past where we were used to fishing for clues to our own and our clients' histories. There were always fat fish to haul up, stuff and display triumphantly over our mantelpiece: "My father drank!" "My mother didn't love me!" "I never got to play the oboe!" But these can be as dead, in terms of how we go forward, as any gamehunters' trophies. Fred knew this, and knew how we all so often used them to keep ourselves out of the dangerous unknown living currents of our future biographies. He knew, too, that dissecting our lives yields as little real knowledge as impaling a butterfly on a pin will reveal to us how it flies. It is the eye of imagination, not the pick and shovel of analysis, that beholds such things. And no point-of-view need be too absurd or outrageous, for it is often from the most unlikely angle that we are granted a sudden and surprising view.

When I ask, for instance; "What comes to me through having cancer in Detroit?" I am amazed at the perceptions this brings. Detroit is Cancer City in a certain way. The immune-system that keeps a body or community flourishing broke down long ago. Unemployment runs high, the neighbourhoods have decayed, crack houses – like tumors – abound. It sometimes seems that guns and drugs are the city's chief industry. The violence and depression conditions here engender is not surprising; the consequence of greed, indifference, denial of community that we are all guilty of to some degree. Its problems have been treated in much the same way as conventional medicine treats the cancer patient; raze the neighbourhoods, obliterate or ignore the unsightly visions of poverty, erect new gleaming structures – numb and unliving as artificial breasts; prostheses to hide the hollow places, the mutilations. Attack the symptoms, but do not seek the forces that might truly heal.

Seeing this, should I not leave immediately? It hardly seems an environment in which I might be healed. But no – to run would be to run from my own malignancies and perhaps, thereby, miss just those elements I need to engender a new level of health. This city is set in a total body of fertile earth and healing waters as the calcified blob in my breast is set in a body that potentially has similar revitalizing powers. More significantly, within the city there are grassroots initiatives that show how the problems and the needs can be addressed. I think of SOSAD (Save Our Sons and Daughters), of FOCUS:Hope, the Mother Waddles Mission. They offer inspiring images of courage, hope, endurance, and practical ways to restore community.

So I have, in Detroit, an image of myself. I see my own shadow reflected back to me; my own violence, greed, apathy, fear, despair. Also an image of the light we can all discover within ourselves that seeks to transform and heal. Our times are cancerous. It is not just bodies which are prey to this disease. In letting this place inform me, I may learn better how to approach my own condition. And, through working with my illness, I may even unlock resources to offer something to the sickness in the world. So I find myself grateful for being here – the city and myself in crisis – and whether or not this is the meaning I'm meant to discover, it feels creative to imagine it that way for now.

Another interesting ramble begins when I question the timing of my illness – this year, not last year or the one to come. Lenny arrived here two months before my diagnosis, (and actually moved the following year to some distance away.) I had someone exceptional, ready and willing to treat me, not to mention Dorothea standing by with my daily syringe! While not so narcissistic as to think that Lenny's sole mission in coming to Detroit was to heal me, the timing was certainly a happy one for me. Even more important, perhaps, is the deep connection we have made between our families and the seeds of a future colleagueship we have sown. Is the cancer a means of bringing us together, not an end in itself?

I look at all the other people I've met as a result of this disease. Some are newcomers; others I've met in new and deeper ways. The exchanges with my parents that I treasure so deeply might not have occurred; the crisis unlocking levels of feeling and ways of sharing that I do not know we knew were there. There have been fine moments too with others closer at hand. I think of fiery little Sarah Owsiany roaring under the table, my radiation parties, Suzanne and I discussing all manner of things over our Mexican dinner in Pennsylvania, my trips to Chicago, even my delicious bargains at the Jewish thrift store! I think of mistletoe, of repulsive hospital waiting rooms, the warm brown gaze of Dr. Martino, of all my friends encircling me. What might still happen as a result of all these moments, all these encounters that cancer has brought me? And not just happen to me, but to everyone else?

For this leads to the second great ingredient so often missing in our reflections; what my illness might mean to others, what impact it has on their lives? I believe to think of one's own crises solely in terms of what they mean to us is the true narcissism – the perpetual self-referral for all life's happenings to which we are still so prone. Others bring me my destiny – are my destiny – and lead me as surely along my path as any steps I might think I am taking by myself. My life is the sum of their influence, or the sum of our interactions; the continual encounter between what lives in me and what meets me on all sides. So then I am the other's destiny, my illness, my choices impact on those who surround me, engage and shape their lives as surely as theirs do mine. This is quite a responsibility! No wonder we often tend to ignore it. But without it, we are truly lost on our journey, for this is one, by whatever routes we go, that we share.

I push through my first feelings of horror and guilt that I've imposed such a burden on my friends and family, to wonder if there could be fruitful consequences for others being with me through this time. Of course there are! Look at the care and compassion they have lavished upon me, the infinite patience, the sheer hard work! Cynthia will get strokes in heaven for all the bushels of spinach she has washed, not to mention her calm attendance through all my vicissitudes. The same goes for Mary-Jo, Francina, dozens of others who each in their different ways have exercised – and assuredly strengthened – their extraordinary virtues on my behalf. My parents have gone way beyond supporting me personally in contributing to Weleda's manufacture of *Iscador* in Britain, thus enabling other patients to receive the benefits. Thus, from each person's center, ripples spread.

We may never know to whom our own may reach. We may never know in what ways, directly or indirectly, we may have touched another's life. But we must know that we are doing so; that our thoughts and deeds have as many consequences for others as they do for ourselves. Kathleen Raine's beautiful words return to me, as I ponder the mystery of our shared lives, our interwoven journeys:

> *"We, the many*
> *Rays from the one centre, each some single course*
> *Must take among the innumerable ways;*
> *Yet could we find that point where all converge*
> *Might interchange heart with heart and thought with thought,*
> *Know others as ourselves, all that he has been*
> *Suffered and done, till we are wise*
> *With all earth's sorrows, and at peace."*

Is this, then, truly what it is all about for all of us? Cancer – or any crisis? All our blundering movements, botched encounters, tormented relationships, painful collisions with self or other? Are they all in some way symptoms of our struggle to go forward till we are wise with all earth's sorrows and, despite or indeed because of this, at peace?

This seems a thought to hold, a question to keep on asking, as I go forward myself. I hear my voice again: "Listen", "Love the earth". Perhaps it is as simple and mighty as that for me. Perhaps I should set aside the maps, search no further for meanings, and simply plunge back on the path that leads me somewhere, and trust that life, not my interior monologues, will teach me all I need to know.

Chapter 16

WINTER

"Oh Winter, ruler of th' inverted year
I love thee, all unlovely as thou seem'st."
— The Task, William Cowper.

The winter has been relatively mild so far. Not Californian of course. Plenty of dirty grey snow. The insides of one's nostrils still freeze together on contact with the open air. But it's not as bad as last year. This is a relief. Keeping warm consistently in Michigan from December to March is no mean feat!

I continue my rituals – the private and the public ones. Cynthia, Rob and Mary-Jo come to dinner once a week. Interesting food combinations that need to cater to my regime, plus everyone else's tastes. We settle for rice and *pesto* more often than not. *Pesto* always brings a happy gleam into Rob's eyes, though Adam looks fairly disgusted and, I suspect, imagines we will soon be sporting shaggy hair and Birkenstocks. After dinner Adam and Rob do manly things, like giggling and taking out golf clubs to do chip shots in the snow. The womenfolk spend an hour studying and trying to improve our meditative life. Plenty of giggles here too. We were not born yogis, that's for sure.

Once a month we go to Point Pelée – whoever is free to come. We promised my mother. An easy promise to keep. Even in midwinter, there's no such thing as bad weather there, though we often don't trust the fact. One Saturday we set forth in freezing rain. Adam grumbles most of the way. "Why are we going?" he asks glumly, repeatedly, as we drive down through the city, over Ambassador Bridge, beneath which the river flows grey, cold, beaten flat by icy sleet.

Yet, when we jog through the thickets, heads down against the wind, and emerge on to the promontory, he gasps and cries: "*Now* I know why we came!" The sand is heaped with ice crystals from end to end. At that moment the clouds part and a pale sun slants down, burnishing them with rainbow hues. A fairy world. We rush into them, burying our legs in piles of jewels – diamond, opal, sapphire – and then fall and roll in them, piling them over each other in great glittering heaps. Never mind that they fill our boots, will melt in icy streams down the back of our necks. A miracle is worth a sodden aftermath, and there are hot cappuccinos awaiting us in a Portuguese pool bar on the way home. Yes, each day spent here is uniquely magical – an astonishing replenishing interlude between weeks spent shored up in the city, amidst the wail of sirens and the various stresses of our daily lives. I sleep with the sound of far off waves, feeling myself gently rising and falling on their ebb and flow.

There are other miracles. I am sure they come daily, but we do not notice them. When I go for one of my check-ups with Dr. Martino, mine for this day is staring me straight in the face. The waiting room is transfigured. The orange, purple and lime green chairs have gone and in their place are some delightful heathery, tweedy ones. Wood frames too, not coldly glittering chrome. And incredibly comfortable. As if this were not enough, the whole area is filled with huge and wonderful plants. After I've given about half my blood to a nurse I rush into my cubicle.
"What's happened?" I ask Dr. Martino. "Has this hospital had a revelation or something?"
She chuckles. "No – that would be too much to hope for. A patient donated them." Well, I suppose it would have to be that. We are the ones who know what harms or heals. I do hope it wasn't a legacy. I'd like to think of her – it is a woman, naturally – getting the benefit, as well as enjoying the pleasure we all must feel. It certainly makes this trip ten times more relaxing. In fact I feel more relaxed than Dr. Martino seems herself today. She looks tired and strained. She admits this when I ask. "Periodic burn-out," she explains. Oh dear, how self-absorbed I've been. I've never once considered what it might be like for her, day after day. I tell her she'd better take good care of herself, but sense this is an unhelpful injunction. To do that she might have to pull out of the system and I don't believe she's prepared to abandon us. Thinking of her, and of Lenny doing his 100-hour hospital week, plus his private practice, I feel there must be a better way for these doctors to exercise their gifts without nearly killing themselves. It certainly isn't good when they look in worse shape than their patients. For the first time I step beyond my own needs and preoccupations to imagine the lives of my healers – and perhaps that's also something of a little miracle.

I actually feel pretty well these days – in better shape too than most of my friends. They are all running their second or third winter cold. Perhaps in this mild winter the bugs don't die off. But I haven't had one yet, and take this as testimony to an improved immune-system. I also feel pretty smug, and offer therapeutic advice to the snuffling company. But then they get the 'flu – and that is accompanied by a FEVER! I am smug no longer. I am pea-green with envy. I want a fever too. Cynthia tells me she's up to 101°. When John's temperature reaches 104° I am ready to do violent things. I listen to pale hoarse voices on the telephone, bring groceries to humped figures lying under heaps of bedclothes, hand glasses of juice into limp hands. "I'm so sorry," I hear myself say in sugary tones, while I fume inwardly. What did they do to deserve this? What must I do to deserve a fever too?
Then one morning I wake with aching bones and a shrieking periphery. I

cringe from contact with the world of objects – the great Untouchable – and spend the day creeping about the house avoiding doorknobs and countertops. I've no idea what's going on, but I crawl around till 4 o'clock when it's time to take my temperature to monitor the *Iscador*. The thermometer reads 102°. I think it must have developed a fault. Surely fevers aren't like this? It is so long since I had one I've forgotten the symptoms, and imagine I'd feel hot and flushed not aching and cold. I take it again. It's still up there. Then the delicious fact really dawns on me. Whoopee! I rush to the telephone to let Dorothea know I can't come for my injection the following day.

"Wonderful!" she says. "Keep warm now."

I call Cynthia – now recovered from her bout with 'flu – to ask her to take care of Adam when he comes home. Then bundle into bed, feeling ecstatic, and cover every square millimeter of myself with heavy blankets. Oh joy, oh rapture – by evening the mercury nearly tips 103°! Lenny even pops in the following day to celebrate. Well, we all have our peak experiences; some on mountain tops, some on the high of romantic love, some on drugs. This is mine; curled up in bed, my body aching and shaking all over, my soul in bliss.

Fevers are seen traditionally in anthroposophic medicine as a chance to make a fresh start. They are welcomed, encouraged to run their course with no outside interference. A parent, new to this approach, might feel understandably upset when calling a doctor to report a child's raging temperature to be met by the response: "That's splendid" and to be told on no account to give aspirin or antibiotics, but simply keep the child warm and look for signs of new development when they are well. The individual is strengthened through the struggle to overcome an illness, and we all too readily deprive ourselves and others of this vital opportunity.

As Philip Incao, an anthroposophical doctor in Harlemville, New York, put it so excellently in an article challenging immunization: "We are so afraid of nature. What is the purpose of our life? If this purpose is to allow our individuality to unfold and express itself to the fullest, then this happens through the process of the immune-system unfolding and reacting as self meets nonself. We become susceptible to infectious disease when we open ourselves to the world. Then we can become full human beings." If we are sensitive, we can usually observe radical changes in a young child after an illness. Often these are striking physical developments: a button nose begins to sprout a beak, limbs shoot out, a threshold to a new motor skill is crossed. In the adult, changes are more inward, psycho-spiritual – that is, if we give ourselves the chance. Adult development is largely a matter of free choice. After an illness we too often scramble to pick up the pieces and give ourselves no time to question if a new element is striving to find a place in our lives. The value of convalescence is no longer recognized as it was a century ago, when at least some socio-economic classes could retreat to spas or seaside resorts. "It is in convalescence," one doctor once told me, "that the Christ can work most particularly." In his language he meant the spirit of transformation and renewal that must inhabit the core of all healing impulses. I was very struck by this comment and tried thereafter to leave space in which I might discover the new element that might await me after an illness.

This fever, then, was not simply a delightful bonus that might have burned off stray cancer cells. Potentially it could unlock energy for a new, creative step. In the lovely cleansed aftermath of a three-day 'flu I attended to what this might be. To my dismay, what came to me was the decision to write.

I have about as many resistances to writing as a porcupine has quills, and these have their history. From the age of six or seven I resolved to be a writer and completed my first novel – by far the best – at the age of nine. By twelve I was writing poetry. In my teens I reverted to novels again. I disliked them all. I suspected others would too. I was aware that I descend from a blood-line of bad novelists. My three maiden great aunts, whose most exotic travels from Yorkshire were their annual trips to London for a Literary Ladies' Luncheon, wrote astonishing romances set in Japanese prison camps or leper colonies in Africa. I admired their courage and ingenuity, their stubborn refusal throughout long lifetimes to drop their pens. But I could not admire the product of their imaginations. And I did not admire the product of mine.

My swansong took place in Italy in my late twenties. I rented a remote watermill in the Tuscan hills with the dual aim of recovering from a long and painful love affair and writing the novel of the century. It seemed at least a hundred other people had the same idea – at least about writing; I cannot speak for their love lives. The hills were dotted with stone cottages, each inhabited by an author. The strains of tap-tapping typewriters mingled daily with cowbells and tinkling streams. One man was on his second book. He'd sold the film rights to the first. Another woman was completing her first slim volume of poetry, already accepted by a publisher. I was absolutely paralyzed, except for a few frivolous pages on how *not* to write a book – the first step being to rent a Tuscan watermill and thereby expose oneself to the frustrating, yet delicious distractions of Italy. I returned to England with neither goal achieved. The love affair still trickled on.

Back home I co-authored some food guides with my friend and author, Judith Thurman, who came to live with me for a while. The pay-off (eating) just about compensated for the sweat over writing about what we ate. I also had, in Judith, an exquisite editor. I'd produce the roughage and she would refine it with copious strokes of her red pen, reducing my reams of raw bulk to a few poetic essences. But it was a struggle nonetheless. At the end of our assignments, Judith asked me point blank: "Do you want to write?" "No," I said. Hearing my voice speak this with such calm certainty was a enormous relief. Until her question I hadn't realized I felt that way. She returned to New York to write a fine biography of Isak Dinesen. After a chaotic interlude I was drawn into the field of psychotherapy.

People's lives were far richer and more extraordinary than any fiction I could dream up. Whatever minimal literary capacities I might have had quickly atrophied, so that I actually dreaded putting pen to paper for almost any reason at all.

With all the forgoing, why would I decide to try again? It seemed a crazy idea. Yet it kept coming back. It came from others too. "Yes," I'd mutter vaguely, when friends suggested it. "Maybe I will one day." I know how often I suggest to others that they write about their experiences. I mean it too. But I suspected that some of my friends thought if I wrote about it, I wouldn't talk about it quite so much. They were probably pretty bored by now. The finer details of mammogram machines and breast injections must be about as interesting as a lesson in how to fold diapers is to the childless. I thought of all those millions of words out there; even the thousands devoted to tales of cancer and miracle cures. What on earth was the point of adding mine?

Despite such reasonable objections, I found myself beginning one day. I decided to write something every day for a year, and then I would stop. Inherent in this plan were two goals: to discipline myself to give form to a year of experience so that I could lay it aside and move on; and to honor some of the people who play a part in it. If they never reached public awareness, I needed to remember them.

Chapter 17

NO-MAN'S LAND

"And when they were only half way up,
They were neither up nor down."
– The Grand Old Duke of York,
English Nursery Rhyme.

I have begun to establish something of a writing rhythm – not daily, of course, but we can't all be perfect – when another Judith comes for a three week visit. This Judith is one of my oldest friends. We first met when I was a nervy, fairly vapid ex-debutante, and she had been recently widowed and was facing the immense task of rearing two children under three. Within six months we were sharing a flat in London. I had begun to work for John Betjeman, (later Poet Laureate,) and Judith had embarked on a teacher training program, her parents kindly caretaking her children while she became professionally qualified.

I was into Poetry, Victorian architecture, and Rich Food (as increasingly defined by John B.) Judith was informed and active in left-wing politics, education and social problems. Apart from humor, a mutual terror of spiders and a predilection for unsatisfactory love affairs, we seemed to have little in common. Yet our friendship flourished. It survived years when our interests ranged even further apart. To Judith's dismay, I became involved both in Jung's psychology and Anthroposophy. Her dismay was entirely appropriate. There is nothing worse than a novice psychologist unless it be a raw recruit to Anthroposophy. I know I bored and infuriated her with my enthusiastic renderings of dreams and glib appraisals of people's psychopathologies. When she had learned to weather my worst excesses in the psychological realm, I proceeded to enter a spiritual one with, to boot, a name few people can even pronounce!

"Don't you dare bend a benign blue gaze on *me!*" Judith declared vigorously, referring to the peculiar, trance-like expression many newcomers to a spiritual discipline affect. Happily, I can't stay benign for long, but I certainly did not know when to keep my mouth shut. A sectarian has been defined as someone who answers questions no-one has asked. For at least a couple of years I was such an offender; doubly so, since I had two systems of thought to champion and evangelize! The hairline scratch on my nose made by the metal end of a tube of Weleda toothpaste, (manufactured by an anthroposophical pharmacy,) which Judith once hurled at me was probably richly deserved!

However, thanks to her immense stubbornness, and an unshakeable affection we feel for each other, our friendship remains, deepened and strengthened by time and all the vicissitudes life has brought us together and apart.

Of course Judith is one of the first transatlantic friends to whom I break the news of my cancer. It is about as hard as telling my parents, and telling her about Steiner and Jung. I am asking our friendship to stand another trial and I wish I were not. However, she replies with such a delicious, bracing optimism that I feel better immediately. Typically, she includes a couple of wicked observations as to possible causes that have me rolling off my living-room couch. She offers to fly over any time. She hates flying too.

I do, in fact, put her off for a while. I feel I need a few months to sort myself out, establish my new rhythms, my new life. I imagine by then I'll be fit and transfigured in ways that will completely accord with our tried and tested friendship. We will then be able to take a harmonious little vacation together.

This little fantasy proves about as unrealistic as imagining I'd be ready to dance a *pas de deux* with Rudolf Nureyev, as we both learned to our bitter dismay. I was neither one thing nor the other. Whatever charm my old self and old ways had held for me and others had vanished, to be replaced by nothing less than sheer nastiness. Judith's presence mirrored self-images that were strange or sickeningly familiar. I could cope with neither and frequently wished she would disappear so I did not have to look at them.

I discovered I was just about ripe for a Trappist monastery – I, whom my friends probably doubted knew the word "introversion", craved total silence and solitude. Each morning after Adam left for school I'd feel the air settle back around me like the soft comforting touch of angels' wings and I wanted to rest, cocooned in their sheltering power until, or even after, his return. I discovered, too, that I actually wanted to write. More accurately, writing was like a sore tooth that nags and preoccupies all one's attention even while wishing it did not. I wanted to huddle over the pain and discomfort, alone with my pencil and pad. And I didn't want to talk, for fear of leaking energies I needed for the forthcoming masterpiece!

Judith's presence engendered all manner of social calls – as well it might. She had lived with me here for half a year. Several people wanted to see her again. People who had never met her, wanted to for the first time. So, in they flock.

I feel full of holes. Anyone entering my space seems to walk straight through or into me. When Lulu visits, she appears like one of her dogs she's so busy painting; large, voracious creatures, with gleaming eyes and snapping teeth, that consume every canvas; ravaging landscapes, people, houses, cans of beans. I live in a permanent panic of being devoured myself – hardly a healthy condition for the hostess of a three-week house guest, particularly one who has flown the Atlantic and surrendered her life and work to be with me!

Though the desire for solitude was not new, its absoluteness stunned me. I seriously doubted if I wanted any part in the human community again, though I knew I owed my life to it.

Probably, as an inveterate extravert, I had simply sprung to the opposite extreme. Had the old elastic of my astral body snapped completely? Or was it strung so tight, it bounced others back? Sometimes I felt encased in stone, at other times loosely held by a rotting string bag. I read and reread *Tree*, by Deena Metzger. *"She is trying to survive the only way she knows, stepping away from despair and defeat, but somehow in doing it, she is stepping toward another place quite as terrible ..."* and: *"She hated the others, hated them all, and wanted only silence, silence, silence and emptiness and freedom from everyone she knew."* This woman had been through it, and lived to celebrate community. Would I ever reach that place? But this was a no-place now, and who could join me there? I felt sick with guilt and shame, yet powerless to change.

Another painful discovery I made was that I didn't want to think. I did not want to wonder, speculate, analyze. Such activities had always formed the basis of our sharing together – long evenings pondering the course of our own and others' lives; personal and world events, all and any phenomena were grist to our mill. Ideas, which included ideas about feelings and actions, were as important to us as our "comfort foods"; Cream Slices, chocolate bars. How many hundred evenings had we spent feasting on both? Now I wanted neither. Particularly I wanted no ideas about my own condition, or our relationship. I wanted just to be – even in this dark no-man's land of unknowing.

This, like my need for solitude, was not new; simply tremendously strong and, as I saw it, quite incompatible with Judith's presence. What do people do together, other than talk and share? What, specifically, do Judith and I do together? By evening, our familiar appointed hour for sitting by the fire and summing up the universe, I only wanted to creep into bed and burrow into oblivion. This is Judith's brightest hour. She's borne the rest of my day gallantly; my trips to Dorothea for my injection, followed by rest; my eurythmy, followed by rest; my endless preparations of juice and food; the occasional client, the laundry, Adam's return from school and the hours spent together on homework, supper, stories, games. Now comes her time and I'm simply not there. Again, I feel horribly guilty and ashamed and resent this bitterly. I feel I am on the run, and I'm honest enough to admit I am probably running less from her than from myself.

Judith wisely loses her temper with me. Though we've weathered enough fights, I like this one as little as others before. But I need her rage, for I'm passive-aggressive and that helps no-one, least of all myself.

"You want our relationship completely on your terms," she storms, as I crouch like an armadillo over the kitchen sink, presenting her a back full of metallic spines.

"And I don't even know what those terms are!" Nor, of course, do I.

"Shit," I mutter savagely into the dirty dishwater. "It would be better if I died." Yes, I even sink that low. But right now that seems the only solution to this terrible *impasse.*

"And why do you want to change?" she wails. "I liked you the way you were."

"Well, I've just got to," I say desperately. "Being how I was is what got me sick in the first place."

"I don't believe it," she says. Nor, entirely, do I. And nor do I see any virtue right now in attempting to change anything. Lord, shouldn't I be on cloud nine, being affirmed as likeable the way I was, and clearly degenerating hourly into a monster that will probably wind up in a Trappist monastery as the only place on earth that might accept my beastliness? But I continue to mutter darkly about my fate, her lack of sympathy, till she flounces out into the garden and we each, alone and aching, have our solitary weep. When she returns, we stare at each other with red-rimmed eyes.

"I'm angry because I'm scared," I say, with perhaps the first touch of real honesty. "And maybe you are too. I don't know where I'm going. I don't know if I'll change, or what I'm trying to change, or what will happen to us if I do. But I've got to go on."

"Well, it can hardly be worse than it is now," says Judith with a damp, wry grin. "I suppose you'd better carry on." We clasp each other vigorously, but the sores remain and are easily rubbed raw again.

In a calmer time, she questions if I am not already healed.

"You go on saying you've got cancer. I'm assuming you haven't; that the cancer was cut out. I need to know which." Again, I feel myself going into an armored crouch.

"It's not that simple," I say.

"Yes, it is. You've either got it or you haven't. You'd better decide."

"It's both," I say defensively. "I had some that was cut out. but that didn't change anything. I could easily get it again."

"Why should you?" Judith has always been quite clear that she thinks the stress of certain relationships has engendered the disease.

"You know what I think caused this. And you needed to get it off your chest. Well, isn't it off now? Haven't you paid the price?" She looks grimly at my lop-sided frontage. "You certainly don't need to go through any more."

A pretty supportive friend! And I'm very grateful for her flattery and certainty. But there is still this persistent sense that I need to imagine cancer to keep me on my growing edge. "Fear guards the threshold to the future," Rudolf Steiner said, and through encountering our fear we may be led to give birth to some new awareness, some new deed. Something like that, I think, is going on. I try to tell her this and it thrusts us back where we were before, both of us angry and afraid.

"I know I came because I needed to see you, see how you were," says Judith on the verge of tears again. "Not just because I thought you needed me."

"And that's what I can't cope with," I tell her. "I can't cope with other people's needs. Right now," I add, with a quite gratuitous brutality, "I feel like sending out a color photograph – "This Is Me Now". I don't want everyone swarming here to satisfy their curiosity as if I were a circus freak."

"We're *not*!" She yells. "And it's *not* everybody! It's just your friends who love
you. Can't you see we need to know how you are?"

And so on and so forth. I see her position far better than I see my own. When
she repeats that she shouldn't have come if I hadn't agreed to it, I have no answer,
no excuse. I simply did not know how I would be. And I wonder if I'll ever know
again. So bang goes any plan with anyone who lives more that half-an-hour away.
Those çlose can clearly scuttle home to lick the wounds I have inflicted on them.

We are obviously wrestling with the clear, yet terrifying dilemma posed by
any shift of ground by one person in a relationship. This is compounded by my
having no ground myself. Judith so often asks me merely to clarify what I want,
so she can adjust to it. But I don't know what I want, or if I will ever know. We
agree it would actually be far easier if I was obviously ill; could lie around wanly
while she ministered. This damn disease is so invisible. Is it secretly eating away
at me? How long, oh Lord, how long must I live this way, hurting my friends and
feeling pain myself? I also begin to realize that I have moved into another phase,
when I can no longer use the cancer, the immediate crisis of surgery, as an excuse
or motive for what I am doing. This is the scariest moment yet.

I feel Judith, both for herself and as a representative of a particular viewpoint,
is asking for an untarnished replica of myself B.C. as a guarantee of my return to
health. And I am seeking some delicious transfiguration as testimony to my
being "better" than I was before. We will surely neither get what we are hoping
for! She shows me, too, how frightening the crises, illnesses of those we care for
are; constellating so many of our own vulnerabilities – fears of loss, fears of
abandonment, simply the fear of any changes in the *status quo*. How much easier
to believe the cancer was a finite, nasty incident, over now and best forgotten, as
we all resume our lives again, rather than something that may change everything.
I half wish I could see it this way, or at least pretend I could. But I am stuck with
this stubborn commitment to something else. There must be *something* if I am
prepared to sacrifice so much for it!

I thank Judith. I tell her I feel thoroughly ashamed, that I still love her, that
I still can't make it easier. I ask her to remember that this visit, coming to its end,
has not been wholly horrible. Remember Easter at Lulu's? Remember our first
Seder with Madalyn? Yes, she agrees, there have been some fine times too.
"Besides," she reflects, as we part at Windsor station, "we've had twenty years
together, and probably have another twenty to go. We can always mark this as
one of the worst holidays we spent. There are surely a few good ones still in store
for us"

I watch her sturdy figure recede, and drive home, feeling quite forlorn, my
eyes misting dangerously as I speed the freeway. My house has a definite hollow
space the shape of Judith which it takes a while to fill again with me.

Chapter 18

INTO THE DARK

"At first the silence is a silence only,
But huge lack bears huge something through the dark"
– The Silence, May Sarton.

I am so appalled by my behavior, and feel so dreadful that after Judith leaves I make a list. I am: *Selfish, Self-absorbed, Stupid, Dark, Confused, Destructive, Violent, Hard, Cold.* What is more, I do not care. I do not care for anyone. I know nothing. I do not want to know. I want to be left alone. I want to do my thing. I do not know what my thing is. I don't want anyone to tell me what it is. I do not want to know.

Sounds like cancer, doesn't it? I don't have cancer. Cancer has me. I am cancer. One large, spreading, malignant blob. Wow! This is the writing on my wall. "I need to look at what is cancerous in my soul," I had told Dr. Martino blithely. I need to look no more. My soul is cancerous from edge to edge. It is taking me over. It is leaking over others, darkening their lives. I am full of fury and a terrible despair. And now I really do feel ill.

My body temperature drops alarmingly. My nerves feel jagged. I have a headache one day in three. None of my therapies alleviate the distress. My gorge rises at the sight of carrot juice. When I do eurythmy, the delicate garment I used to feel around me is tattered and torn. I can feel my limbs poking through the holes. I want to drink five gallons of coffee and smoke a dozen cigarettes. A slug of brandy might be nice, with a steak and french fries. When I break my diet, I feel worse. I can't even enjoy bad food anymore! This is the final bitter irony. Never again to be comforted by a Cream Slice? My God – what will then call me back from the abyss?

The night of my diagnosis, I had had a dream. *"I tell my surgeon, Pamela, that the cancer patient can experience the backside of matter."* The dream is objective, very matter of fact. I found it reassuring at the time. Well, another rich experience, I thought. I now see I'm somewhere in the backside of me, and it's far from rich, unless this stinking mess can be so called. "Garbage is also fertilizer" comments James Hillman. Yes, I agree. But the compost heap in my own garden resolutely refuses to break down, metamorphose into new rich soil. Year after year it reveals thick wooden stalks, globs of congealed orange peel, eggshells, lengths of string, all embedded in a curious ashen substance from which no phoenix could ever rise. And despite all the techniques I follow, the

99

applications of lime, bonemeal, organic unguents, remains unchanged – a perpetual metaphor for my inner life. So what hope for personal resurrection, if I can't turn two cubic feet of leftovers into fertile earth?

I tackle this phase in roughly the same way as I do my gardening. I know no other. I sit and rot. I let the feelings come: grim, bitter, malevolent. Like the Dead Sea, to which I once travelled, this place is desolate – a place of thickening silence too deep for air or life or sound. This is the true interior – a twilight valley of salt, grey ash, dry bones.

I do what I have to do. Eat and sleep. I barely leave the house. I almost never drive a car. I almost never laugh. Except grimly – reflecting how typical of me that it's taken so long to feel so bad. Were all the previous months of cheer and optimism so much illusion? And only now are my defences against reality crumbling?

Dorothea continues to inject my breast. I scuttle home afterwards, afraid to admit my despair. Perhaps the mistletoe is a big hoax? Eurythmy still brings no relief, though I do it doggedly each day. Even bundled under my woolly rugs I feel fragmented and cold. At painting, my colored blobs are heavy, mineralized.

Eve suggests many things. Am I rubbing my body with enough oils? Of course we're full of holes, she says. That's part of it. "I don't understand," I wail. "Dozens of people just keep going – through chemo, through radiation, through much worse surgery. Why should I feel so terrible?"

"We're trying to create another body," she says. "A spiritual body, not just a physical one." Eve always has these grand, strange concepts that I barely understand, wonder if apply to me, yet somehow comfort me.

"What happens if we don't get this 'spiritual body' together before the physical one collapses?"

"Then we'll die," she says cheerfully. "Well, we'll die anyhow. This is for the next life." Next life? I can't even manage next Wednesday. In her rosy space I mind less, though. We're together in this, lugging our tattered remnants, our nutty little half-germinated seeds from here to eternity.

Back home, the hopelessness settles in again. I weep. Frequently. For no obvious reasons. Sluggish salt tears that refresh as little as the Dead Sea itself in which I bathed those many years ago and emerged equally grimy, oily and dead beat.

Sheila writes with her usual timing. "You may be going through an intensive process of discharge for all we know . . . shedding the residue of what you've had to endure these past years. Who knows, the field of cancer may need befriending as well as inhabiting – something to do with Beauty and the Beast." I don't know, but I try to befriend this beast; dark and snarling, or simply cold, withdrawn, inert. In Cocteau's movie, the Beast provided Beauty with glorious dinners. I stoically continue to stir my pots of brown rice and drink my carrot juice.

I put Sheila's black candle on my mantelpiece. She sent it from some shrine dedicated to a saint who claimed to have seen the shadow side of God. I do not light it. I can kindle no flame within myself.

Slowly through these days I begin to accept that this encounter with cancer is a marriage, not a brief affair. A path of commitment to what the disease brings. There's no turning back, yet nothing can be left behind. How I would dearly love to cast off my shadow. But no way. Or not that way, it seems, for me.

> *"Life's remade,*
> *With shovel and spade.*
> *Each dull day*
> *And each despairing act*
> *Builds up the crags*
> *From which the spirit leaps . . ."*

I chant Philip Larkin's lines, a melancholy liturgy, as I sweep the floors and hang the washing out. No spirit leaps in me. Just a dreary succession of grey days.

Cynthia and Mary-Jo are comforting. Mary-Jo knows her own dark hours. Cynthia is so solid and calm. She somehow communicates that there may be a way through, though we seldom speak of this. She is ever practical, and suggests the three of us spend a weekend at her parents' empty house in western Michigan. Certainly better than staying at home. So we bundle up; winter woollies, veggies, medicines, and set forth across the snowy plains. We rent comic movies for the VCR, cook huge amounts of food, regress to adolescence; lolling on sofas, sharing fantasies, even once measuring and comparing our waists and hips.

Walking alone each day for hours upon the frozen lake, I see the trees stark and skeletal, yet still erect, spreading their leafless branches wide and strong into the icy air. They haven't given up. Someone told me their sap begins to rise on the day of the winter solstice. They can't know or feel this yet. But they're prepared to wait for it to surge inevitably into their fingertips. Some have carried their buds all winter through. What an image of stubborn hope. I touch some little crimson ones and tell myself my sap may be rising too, though I feel nothing yet. We have many winters and many springs. I'm glad we came.

A week or so after this I have a dream. *"I am going to meet God. I feel deep awe and fear, but the pull of His presence draws me into Him. As I enter, I experience Him as Darkness, Immensity, Weight."*

The dream stays with me for many days and slowly, from it, perhaps from all this time, I feel myself emerging with a subtle, stronger sense of shape. And I decide to go to Arlesheim, as if this nightly inward journey has prepared me for a very different outer one.

Chapter 19

SPRING

"Now the green blade riseth
From the buried grain,
Seed that in the dark earth
Many months has lain.

Fields of the heart
That dead and bare have been . . .
Love is come again
Like wheat that springeth green."
　　　　　　　　　　　　　　　－ French hymn.

Arlesheim is a small town in Switzerland that hosts two anthroposophical clinics; one – the Ita Wegman Klinic – is general; the Lukas Klinic is specifically for cancer patients. I'd known of both for many years and had wondered about going from the start of this thing. Dr. Fried had encouraged me to do so if I had the chance. My parents had offered to meet the costs. But I'd put this idea, along with so many others, on my backburner – already crowded with pots labelled "spiritual healing", "proper visualization", "macrobiotic diet". When in doubt do nothing, seems to be my motto and I couldn't generate enough enthusiasm, despite Marjanna telling me how much she had enjoyed her own time there, and my knowing I could have the full, unadulterated anthroposophical treatment that I could not hope to get elsewhere. Perhaps that was part of it. Maybe I didn't want to be deprived of my delicious defections, even those moments when I forget I have cancer and imagine I am some regular healthy person leading a regular healthy life.

I did make some tentative enquiries soon after Christmas, writing the Ita Wegman Klinic, which was where Marjanna had gone. For some reason I pictured the Lukas Klinic as dark, heavy, pregnant with gravity. I imagined it full of the kind of seriousness I was not yet prepared to feel about my disease. I saw operating, rather than luncheon tables, nasty instruments, hospital smells. It made me think of boarding school; cold stone, linoleum polish, military dormitories. Almost better to die! According to Marjanna the Ita Wegman Klinic was friendly and comfortable, an old house set in flowery gardens. She was even able to tell me what she had for lunch. I need this kind of tangible reassurance when stepping into the unknown.

They replied to my enquiry in German. This was rather discouraging, since the only word I know is "Auf wiedersehen" and that was absent from the literature. A friend translated, but this was just the setback I needed to give it no further thought.

In my new mood of determination, I call Marjanna again. She reassures me immediately. Nearly everyone spoke English there. The benefits were hard to describe, but she had enjoyed her visit immensely. Why had she chosen this place, rather than the Lukas Klinic? She wasn't entirely sure. Her family had a long-standing connection with the former and she had met people there that, with hindsight, confirmed her in her choice. What mine should be, neither of us had any way of knowing. I asked her if she had seen the Lukas Klinic while she was there. No, she hadn't. It grew darker in my imagination, shunted down an alley, perhaps only to be attended by those whose illness was so advanced that a general clinic lacked the resources to handle it. Marjanna said she'd heard only that the clinics were quite different, in structure and content. There was a quite special approach at the Lukas Klinic designed to meet the needs – psycho-spiritual as well as physical – of the cancer patient. I felt lumped into a general category by this thought; stripped of my uniqueness, and horribly visible to the searing gaze of doctors and therapists. The typical Cancer Personality all over again. By comparison, the Ita Wegman Klinic grew rosier though, knowing Arlesheim to be a small town, I had fantasies of being hauled out of my bed there and dragged to the Lukas Klinic where I properly belonged. I guess in anxious moments we do regress, but my infantile attitude to this whole question shamed me vigorously, as it always will.

Plucking up my courage, I phoned the Ita Wegman Klinic to see if they had room, first grappling with continental directory assistance, full of rapid German. Oh God, I thought as I waited for a response over the crackling wires. I cut across the first words frantically:

"Do you speak English?"

"Oh yes. How can I help you?" The voice was a woman's, light and musical. I had a vivid picture of Switzerland: neat, orderly, the mountains, the valleys, the sturdy villages; pretty, prim, trim, above all, safe. Far more familiar to me than the strange spaces of this country I now inhabit. I felt an unexpected longing prick behind my eyelids. How had I imagined I belong here? America is truly the most foreign place on earth to me. A host of anguished feelings rise as we continue to talk. Yes, I definitely need to go to Europe. I need to breathe familiar air again, to be carried by what I know, into which I can insert myself as snugly as a baby strapped to its mother's back. The stress of grappling day by day with a nature and culture that is so alien must be relieved, if only for a few weeks. I imagine Switzerland as one might imagine breathing oxygen again after years of inhaling other substances. Maybe, as much as anything else, living here had ground down my resistances to this disease. Even if not, I need the uplift now.

The woman tells me they could accommodate me through the dates I have in mind. I thank her, and say I'll let them know. Put down the phone and, yes, have a good cry. Her voice still echoes in my ears like a bell summoning me.

I'm just about set to confirm with them, when Eve says casually: "Why wouldn't you go to the Lukas Klinic?" I don't have a good reply. She's never raised this question before.

"It is *the* cancer clinic. If anyone knows anything about this disease, it's them. And Dr. Rita Leroi would be there." She tells me about Dr. Leroi, for whom she once cleaned house. She is one of the greatest doctors in this field. She has a reputation that extends far beyond the clinic and the enclaves of anthroposophical medicine. She travels and lectures the world over. She and her late husband founded the clinic some twenty years ago. Interesting how these facts have never emerged before. Eve goes off and returns with bundles of literature. There are even a few photographs; of Hiscia, the research center; a patient lying in a deep wooden bath, another being tenderly wrapped in sheets of beeswax. One shows some young men suspended fifty feet up a snow-laden pine tree gathering mistletoe in heavy cotton bags. I am intrigued. More than that, as I pour over all this, I am profoundly moved. The descriptions speak of a deeply sensitive human engagement with this illness and the people who bear it. Surely I cannot pass up this opportunity?

I wake up next morning knowing clearly that this is where I want to go; although I am still afraid, of being a patient, of going into something really quite unknown. And I am more afraid of not being accepted, as I begin the process of negotiation; sending my pathology reports, checking dates for available space that coincide with care for Adam and the rest of our summer plans. It is all finally arranged. My request for two weeks is accepted by the clinic, with the response that "if you could stay a little longer, we think we could help you more." I change it to three. The die is cast.

Now I notice the spring. It has crept upon me unawares. Perhaps now that my juices are flowing, I can see and feel them in the world around.

Waxy greenish flowers unfurl on my little dogwood tree. Scarlet tulips appear in unexpected places. The serrated leaves of poppies, the red spears of peonies begin to break through the softening winter crust. Sometimes I lie on my bed, the window framing a creamy foam of pear blossom, and I say a prayer that I may know which is to be my last spring on earth so I can be sure to find a pear tree wherever I am at such a time. Though perhaps, watching the apple blossom – pink and white – beyond, I could make do with that.

Now I can dig, get my hands well under. I don't think we were meant to stay only on the surface of this world. We need to go deeper, feel roots, moist worms, rich crumbly soil. Puttering, planting, pruning, I am very happy these days.

There are strange signs of my own renewal too. When I go to get my hair cut down the street, José looks surprised.

"Back so soon?" she asks.

"Well, it does seem to have got rather out of hand."

"Let's see what it needs." José whisks about, her thoughts as agile as her fingers, telling me about her recent paintings, her enrollment in *A Course of Miracles*. She interrupts herself to run a tuft of my hair through her hands.

"Much thicker," she comments. "I'm going to have to shape it quite a bit today. And it has grown fast." Checking her book, she tells me it is less than three weeks since I last came.

Well, I am impressed. Though my hair will still be thinner than most people's and the grey is still overtaking the brown, I count this a great achievement. I've no idea whether three tons of brown rice, or antimony or eurythmy can take the credit, but it is a pleasant surprise.

Another awaits me at the dentist. Georgia cleans my teeth and pronounces the oral situation to be better than a year ago.

"How's the bite guard?" asks Dr. Grodin, popping in to check me out.

"Bite guard?"

"Yes. We made you one last year."

"My gosh! I forgot about that. I only wore it a couple of times."

"No more trouble then?" No, clearly not. How extraordinary! I had this thing made, in desperation and at great expense, when my perpetual toothache was seen to be caused by my grinding my jaws so fiercely at night that the roots of my lower molars were being continually bruised. I must have stopped grinding. And I can only believe that some combination of medicaments, therapies, vegetarianism has actually had a calming effect. I tell Dr. Grodin. He raises his eyebrows, but comments: "I guess that could be it." The bite guard is, sadly, not refundable. But perhaps that's just as well. This costly piece of plastic can adorn my bathroom shelf as a reminder that, whatever else still seeks transformation, one slight improvement has been made.

Lenny tells me I look ten years younger. Like me, he exaggerates, so let's make it five. Of course anyone who has slept as much and done so little should see a few years fall away. I feel it is time to take up a few dropped activities, or I might regress to a totally irresponsible infancy. The world seems to think so too. I begin to get invitations to give talks or workshops further afield. This involves overnights, travelling. And I feel a surge of panic, even though I accept. Who will inject me? How do I transport my medicines in the increasing heat? What will I eat? My first trip to Ann Arbor answers these questions promptly. Mary-Ann, with whom I am staying, tells me she's happy to inject the *Iscador*.

"I used to give Timur his asthma shots," she says, scooping aside her history books and setting up the surgery. Her fridge is full of fresh vegetables. I only have to add my bag of brown rice. Two people on the workshop say they would have injected me had I asked. Two others offer to do it on Adam's school camping trip. I enter a culture I didn't know existed, where one in five women know how to handle such things. And they've learned, not from the drug scene, but from the exigencies of family life. For a month or more I avail myself of their expertise, happily baring my breast to any stranger prepared to wield a syringe. I only have to transport food and medicines in a natty little insulated bag, but more often than not a hostess or organizer is standing by with a juicer and a mound of organic vegetables.

I do feel, however, that I must learn to inject myself by the time I travel to England. Though my mother has done some pretty amazing things for me in her life, this task is not one I am going to ask of her. She used to pass out when I had shots in childhood, once found in a crumpled heap in the doctor's waiting room. I've no sooner made this resolve, when Dorothea says she'll be away for a few days in a couple of weeks' time. She's going to an Indian Pow Wow in northern Michigan.

"I've worked out that I'll miss one day of your cycle," she says. "By the way, Howard has offered to do it. He mentioned this a long while ago. He wanted to be a back-up if you needed him. I don't know how you feel about this?" Feel? Deeply, gratefully moved; that Howard would have thought about this and tactfully conveyed his concern to Dorothea all those months ago. Howard is a dentist. A breast or a gum, I'm sure it's all the same to him. It is to me too, and it is not coyness on my part that refuses his kindly offer. I just think this is the opportunity I have been fearfully waiting for.

Dorothea sets forth, the car crammed with five children, tents, baby's bottles, on a six-hour journey in blazing heat. I carry home my trivial load: Syringe, vial, alcohol pad. Whose is the greatest ordeal, I wonder, as I fall asleep that night, imagining her setting up camp amidst the tent caterpillars, wailing babies, pounding drums?

In the morning, my own heart pounding, I set things up for myself. Reading glasses, flat surfaces, a cup of coffee to steady my nerves. It takes all of twenty minutes to fill the syringe. The moment that is done, I clutch a fold of my breast and, eyes shut, shoot as fast as I can. Take a deep breath, wait till my trembling subsides. Then, as I sit there, a cold horror washes over me. I forgot to take the air bubbles out! Oh, God. That means I'm about to die. I feel faint, and want to put my head between my knees. No, don't do that. The bubble might reach my brain quicker that way. I sit, rigid, in my chair. Adam is in his room. Shall I call him at once, and speak my last fond memorable words? The minutes pass. How long will it take? At that moment the telephone rings.

"Answer it, will you," I call weakly to Adam through pinched lips. He pounds downstairs.

It's Karen," he yells. Well, perhaps I'd better risk a move. Karen might be able to help. If not, at least I can warn her of my imminent demise. I walk very very slowly down the stairs, clutching the bannisters and feeling quite odd.

"Yes," says Karen, not very comfortingly. "I remember having to take the bubbles out. You push up the end of the syringe till you get a drop at the end of the needle."

"I know *that*," I say shrilly. "But that's what I forgot to do. What happens now?"

"I don't know," she says. "Have you got a copy of Dr. Spock?"

"No. Of course not." I'm beginning to feel quite angry and, as a result, far less faint.

"I could go to the library for you," she suggests doubtfully. "But it would take rather a long time."

"I'd probably be dead by then," I say. Then I suddenly begin to giggle. Hysteria, poor girl. Karen catches it too.

"You don't sound as if you're dying," she says, when we recover. "Why don't I ask Paul. See if he knows anything." The minutes tick by. Yes, I certainly feel better, and nearly half-an-hour has passed since I administered the lethal dose of oxygen. Perhaps if I last an hour I'll live. Karen returns.

"Sorry to be so long. Paul was miles away. And he wasn't much help. He said 'tell her she'll float much better if we go swimming today'".

We giggle again, still slightly hysterical. We make some swimming plans – contingent upon my survival, of course. Karen says she'll call back in half-an-hour, agreeing the bubble couldn't take longer to circuit my bloodstream.

"Thanks," I say. "And Adam will call you if anything untoward occurs." But it doesn't, happily.

When Dorothea returns she tells me I was safe all the time. A very large bubble would have to enter a major artery – well nigh impossible via a subcutaneous injection into the fatty tissue of the breast. And, in the end, her ordeal – known ever after as the Awful Wow Wow – far exceeded mine, with baby Lauren getting third-degree sunburn, the tent caterpillars being far more prolific than even I imagined them, and the ritual dances they'd gone so far to see never actually taking place!

Through all these delights and terrors – perhaps the nature of spring to harbor them – I continue to plan my trip.

"What are you going to wear?" asks Mary-Jo. We look at each other, grinning guiltily. When preparing a workshop together, we can give no attention to form or content until we have planned our wardrobe, down to the last accessory. I go over to her apartment and try on a lot of her clothes. We wind up with my taking off my own shirt, washing it and ironing it dry for her to take to a conference.

"What do people wear to a clinic?" I ask. "I can only think of *Dark Eyes*." In this recent movie, Marcello Mastroianni behaved in his customary outrageous manner amidst a flock of delicious ladies clad from head to foot in white; ruffles, pearl-buttoned bodices, lacy parasols. My image is struck in the 1890s and I have to remind myself we're in the 1980s now. Patients probably wear polyester tracksuits. They probably wear the kind of clothes I wear myself!

Lulu, however, feels it's important to play the part, and unearths a very large, crushed, floppy straw hat.

"Perfect," she says, jamming it on my head. "You look lovely." I'm sure I do. It's at least five sizes too big and has settled down firmly over my nose. Gazing into its dark interior, I tell her I don't want to break a leg, fumbling my way blindly through the Swiss Alps.

"Well, they'll treat you for that too," she tells me blithely. "You can get everything wrong with you while you're there. I'm sure they won't charge extra."

Karen offers further food for thought. "Perhaps you'll meet someone there." She means romance. I giggle.

"What – some elderly German gentleman, dying of cancer?"

"Well, you never know." That's true enough. After all, I'm an aging British woman with the same disease. But it's hardly my idea of an erotic fantasy – a passionate liaison between blood tests and fever baths!

"Doesn't have to be German," pursues Karen, who knows I have some pretty silly ideas about that national character. "Could be Swiss. Or even Dutch." We agree the Dutch are the best. But I still can't conjure up romance. It has not been high on the recent list of priorities. My powers are far too feeble to envisage the Lukas Klinic hosting such an event for me. I return to the theme of my wardrobe, selecting purposeful walking shoes, skirts with elastic waists.

Before I know it, term has ended, the garden planted, and Adam and I are boarding the plane for England where I'll drop him off with my parents on my way to Switzerland and the next stage of this adventure.

Chapter 20

MECCA

"Would it not be a far better method of healing to summon from the depths of man's being, not those forgotten realms which make him ill, but those which make him well, the real spiritual worlds?"
  – The Three Years, Emil Bock.

"You like to have this apple?" A smiling, pink-cheeked nurse's aide holds out the fruit in the palm of her hand.

An apple? I've just staggered up from a kingly feast. In an hour or so I'll be brought Swiss crispbread and fruit tea in case I don't make it through to a supper of fragrant soup, salads, fresh-baked breads, continental cheese. My second bowl of muesli, full of red currants and creamy yoghourt lies untouched since breakfast, and every surface that isn't filled with flowers holds bowls and saucers of local fruits.

"No room," I say, patting my belly which rises beneath the bedclothes as incontestable evidence.

"But it is *si jolie*. Look!" I do look. It is *jolie*; a Snow White apple, red and yellow cheeked. She puts it in my hand, smiles and departs. I carry it to my sun-filled balcony and look at it as if I never saw this fruit before. Red and gold it lies, filled with that same sun that slants down upon the distant, wooded Jura hills. Below in the garden stands the apple tree, its branches hosting that other fruit; round thriving clumps of mistletoe, filled with berries green and white. Birds chatter among its leaves. One, curious, flutters to the edge of my balcony, alights and looks at me with bright, enquiring eyes.

"What's going on?" it seems to ask, as well it might. What, indeed, is happening here?

I arrived at the Lukas Klinic about 4 o'clock on a Saturday afternoon. I could have been earlier, but I funked it at Basel and spent a couple of hours at the railway station, drinking tea and reading an English novel. Once I was there, there was no escape; no fooling myself or others that I was merely on vacation. But eventually I boarded the local train, filled with Italians, and let it carry me out through the suburbs, running through steep wooded cuttings and along the backs of neat gardens full of flowers and vegetables, with the occasional cow tethered beneath a widespread cherry tree. Yes, this is Switzerland: compact, orderly, every square inch meticulously clean and cultivated, the window-boxes brimming with geraniums between brightly painted wooden shutters and, here and there, a vineyard or cornfield angling up the lower slopes of the hills, many of which are crowned with a small castle whose ramparts or tower can briefly be glimpsed above the trees.

At Dornach I took a cab and the driver swirled me the last mile or so with such speed that I barely took in my surroundings. A general impression of flowers blooming over garden gates. Then he swept into the driveway and I got out. I took a deep breath; then a few more, adjusting to the reality that now replaced my earlier vision of an old, cold hospital down some dark alleyway.

I stood in front of a long low peach-colored building. Scarlet awnings shaded little terraces. Large windows reflected sunlight. Flowers bloomed at the feet of flowing sculptures. A great mural of a figure with the staff of Mercury and a winged bull covered one wall. At the entrance the branch of mistletoe, shaped like a chalice, was emblazoned. I could smell the roses that arched over the doorway. I picked up my luggage and walked in.

A friendly young man at reception greeted me. I remembered his voice from one of my transatlantic calls. Within seconds a nurse appeared, speaking excellent English, and took me down broad, sunny corridors to my room. "We said you would have to share a room for the first days, didn't we?" She asked. "I hope you don't mind."

I can hardly complain. The corner room is large and airy, with an inviting little balcony set with two comfy chairs. The walls, moulded at the corners to give the impression of being inside a crystal rather than a cube, are watercolor-washed a soft, transparent apricot. There are gold curtains at the windows, a soft blue cotton drape dividing the space between the beds. The honey-colored furniture – closet, desk, easy chairs – is carved in soft planes. The beds are piled high with crisp white cotton down comforters. Every surface holds vases of fresh, brightly colored flowers. When I have unpacked and am waiting for my doctor to come and meet me, I go out on the balcony and look across the view to the Jura hills. Right below stands a single apple tree, bearing its dark-leaved clusters of mistletoe – the symbol and reality of this place.

Being too often prone to instant judgements that oppose reality, the next couple of hours give me plenty of cause for shame. First, my doctor arrives. He's at least fifteen years younger than me. He has a beard and wears Birkenstocks. Despite his white coat, my file, and some official-looking objects in his breast pocket, he looks innocent and uncertain, and I immediately assume, by arriving on a weekend, I have been delegated to some untried intern and my life and fate now lie in less than capable hands. We spend about an hour together. Adjusting to the English language, his questions and comments sound tentative. It takes me about half that time to recognize they are, in the best possible sense. It is slowly conveyed to me that Dr. Riggenbach is creating an open space in which we may both begin to form a relationship. Moreover, this space is surrounded by warmth; his warmth, held quietly on the periphery. It does not intrude, and it takes me a while to feel its presence. In fact, it takes several meetings to see this for what it is. But even in this first hour, a truth knocks on the door of my conscience; a truth brought in many ways and forms, by many people, during the next three weeks, that I begin, at first with some discomfort, to ingest. It is a truth about love.

Along with an initial "getting to know me", Dr. Riggenbach outlines some general procedures and explains it will take several days to create my individual program of therapies. He seems particularly concerned that I suffer no anxieties through the weekend when therapy is suspended, and plans to talk with me again the following day. He gives me a long, quite fascinating biographical questionnaire to fill in at my leisure. When he leaves, I go back over our interview. I feel I could have told him many things I did not. I brought some burning questions with me – and not a few clever and interesting observations too! There was nothing in his manner to suggest he would be unreceptive to anything I wished to declare. It is just that somehow the questions burn a little less intensely, the comments feel less clever and less interesting now. I take out my copy of Parzival to read until suppertime.

The second cause for a proper humbling comes in the person of my fellow patient, Frau Gantz, who returns shortly after from an outing with her family. She is a German woman, in her sixties I would guess; painfully thin, but walking erect on her husband's arm. Her skin is a sallow yellow, so are the whites of her eyes. She and her company greet me warmly in German and, when they realize I don't understand them, attempt a few words of English.
"I spik only a little little Inglisch," says Frau Gantz, smiling sadly and apologetically, as her husband helps her into bed. She hardly needs to apologize when I can only say "*Ja*" and "*Auf wiedersehen*". I shrug and sigh and smile back.

Well, I had my little fantasy of sharing a room with an elderly German woman. And so I am. But the difference is that I had imagined a tough, large-breasted, somewhat military figure, fierce and whiskery as my German teacher at boarding school, barking incomprehensible orders at me while I scuttled about seeking a little private space. And here is a woman who only had to look at me with those warm brown eyes and her regretful smile, to have found a place in my heart.

A muted gong summons us to supper and I follow figures emerging from doorways, moving down the spacious shallow stairway, illumined by great watercolors of the painting school Eve attended, till we converge on the dining room. A crisp figure awaits us to show us to our places.
"Ah, Frau Sturgeon-Day," she says, smiling warmly. "Welcome. You are at the top table. There will be people who speak English there."
I find my place, set with an embroidered napkin holder bearing my name, and

look about to get an impression of my fellow-patients. They seem to come in all shapes and sizes, men and women, covering a broad range of ages, and stages of this disease. One has crutches, a few are supported on the arms of friends. Two or three are hauntingly young. Others, like myself, seem hearty and hale. On the whole this might be anywhere; a quality hotel in the Swiss mountains, but a rather unique one, with the soft golden furniture, the ceiling washed in turquoise and cobalt veils of color, some intriguing planetary forms cast in different metals ornamenting one wall. And, of course, flowers everywhere; glimpsed through the great windows, making a vivid centerpiece on each damask tablecloth. At an unspoken signal, the low murmur of voices ceases and we bow our heads to receive the Grace, spoken in German, the English words of which I know so well.

> *"The plant-seeds are quickened in the night of the Earth,*
> *The green herbs are sprouting through the might of the Air,*
> *And all fruits are ripened by the power of the Sun.*
>
> *So quickens the soul in the shrine of the Heart,*
> *So blossoms Spirit-power in the light of the World,*
> *So ripens Man's strength in the glory of God."*

Together we bless the meal, greet each other and begin: soup, full of aromatic herbs, served from a great silver tureen; a crisp pie of cheeses and fresh vegetables topped with roasted sesame seeds, large bowls of salad in a creamy dressing, followed by larger bowls of fruit – raspberries, red currants, peaches, and the big black cherries for which the Swiss are renowned. This is a far cry from my single platter of brown rice and vegetables. I am a little aghast, and refuse the dessert. "Is there something else you would prefer?" asks the server solicitously.
"Oh no. I'm just very full."
"Well, take some with you. You might want it later." Thus begins, even at this first meal, the stockpiling against a siege that never comes!

I learn from my table companions that they will be going to a eurythmy performance tonight at the Goetheanum, but that it is too late to get a ticket for me. There will, however, be a concert at the clinic as there is every Saturday night. I thank them and say I may just go the bed. We discover where we have come from: Switzerland, Germany, France, Australia, South Africa. I am the only patient from America. We ask about each other's lives, work, family. It is a rule, my neighbor explains, that we do not speak about our disease at meals. By the time we rise, I feel I already have friends. One expresses the hope that I will not feel lonely tomorrow – Sunday – which many will spend with their families. I return to my room, feeling far from alone, and quite glad now of my semi-private space. Frau Gantz is already in bed. I sit a while on the balcony and then, too, undress. I am tired now and, before it is fully dark, fall asleep to the strains of a Bach sonata being played downstairs.

After a delicious breakfast in bed, Dr. Riggenbach returns. The only treatment or therapy on this day of rest is our injection of *Iscador*, administered in our abdomens. He explains the effects will be closely monitored so that the most effective dosage can be found before I leave. I must take my temperature rectally every two hours. Blood tests will be given once a week. I will need to have a chest X-ray and an abdominal ultrasound. I don't like the sound of this. I am reminded that this is not just a delightful vacation, easy enough to pretend, lying in bed, full of freshground coffee and bread rolls, with the sun streaming through the window and the birds singing in my apple tree. But today is Sunday. I am free to do as I please, which is now to forget X-rays and go out to explore this place, my home for the next three weeks.

I dress and go into the town. Walking up narrow streets I discover an enchanting world of small, close-set houses, huddled up slopes, intersected by narrow alleys, some paved with cobblestones. The deep tiled roofs glow in the sun. Window boxes full of flowers abound. It is like entering a fairytale; gnomes and elves are surely hiding in the clumps of gigantic cowparsley, a witch or princess sitting high up in one of these attic rooms. The few shops are closed. What a relief! I've never got used to America; its dishonoring of any day of rest or festival; the malls brimming on Sundays; stores proudly announcing their hours for Christmas and Easter Day. We need these quiet hours to withdraw from the seductions of the material world, perhaps to enter another dimension of reality. This town certainly sets the scene for alternative experiences.

I move on, beyond the houses, following a path beside meadows full of slender, large-eyed, coffee-colored cows. As they eye me and move away, the bells around their necks ring out a medley of notes. And, as if in answer, the bells from all the churches begin to chime. The air is filled with interweaving harmonies, deep and low, compelling and clear, calling all to worship, from cottage, house and farm. Then, abruptly as it began, the music ceases and an infinite quietness falls over the land. I pause under a great beech tree, bowing my head for my own moment of silent prayer, inhaling the acrid smell of last year's rotted leaves, hearing close by the soft chatter and gurgle of a little stream. What a place, I think, an hour later, as I wander slowly home. I feel the healing here has already begun without a single official therapy.

Sunday lunch is a splendid festival. Some patients are missing – their places taken by husbands, wives, friends and children of the remaining ones. The room resounds with merry chatter. The meal – four courses – is a triumph of culinary art. In all my days as a food writer I seldom saw, or tasted, anything to compare. After months of relative asceticism, I pick my way gingerly through the various delights and again refuse dessert which, to my amazement, includes ice cream – one of the great "No-No's" of the anthroposophical cancer diet. I ask my neighbor about this; a pretty young woman with a merry laugh, whom I've learned is here for the third time, finally sending her disease into remission, feeling it gradually recede from lung and bone.

"Oh," she says, "so many patients are not used to this diet. They miss their steaks and *pommes frites*. So, on Sundays they get a little treat."
"Aren't they familiar with this approach?" I ask. I had supposed all patients were sent by anthroposophical doctors and were well indoctrinated in vegetarianism and all else besides. My companion corrects this notion immediately. It seems the majority are quite new to this treatment, having been referred by local surgeons and oncologists. "This place has a great reputation," she informs me. "Often patients come here, too, when everything else has failed."

This impresses and intrigues me. What must some patients think? I can see from the several flat or lopsided chests, the number of wigs, that many have had considerable exposure to surgery, radiation and chemotherapy. I wonder what they make of a painless abdominal injection, a few genial physical and artistic therapies? I must ask them in the coming days. But right now it is all I can do to stagger up to my room for a rest before walking over to Dornach to see the Goetheanum. A passing nurse agrees that that will make a fine outing and tells me there will be no "liver compress" today so I am free to go when I like. I haven't a clue what a liver compress is, but I'll surely find out when the weekly rhythm begins. Lovely though this day had been, and continues to be until, full of good food, fresh air and many wonderful sights, I clamber beneath my down comforter again, I am really looking forward to the working week ahead.

In the morning we are awakened by the flute. I think perhaps I have died in the night and am now in Paradise. But I open my eyes to the familiar contours of my room; the sun peeking through gold curtains and patterning the apricot walls. Snug and secure beneath the bedclothes, I can still hear that delicate haunting melody as it recedes down the corridor. I ask Mary-Thérèse, when she comes to draw back the curtains, take my vital statistics and enquire how I slept. "Yes. We were taught in anthroposophical nursing school that the patient should always be woken by music. It helps, you know, to come from night to day." It certainly does. I am perky, ready for breakfast here in this new home, while knowing another as surely awaits me across the threshold of sleep. Some nursing school! There aren't too many of those around, I think.

Slowly this day and following days unfold. Like observing a great painting many times, sometimes I notice the background; the broad landscape receding into hazy, then invisible distances. Sometimes I am aware of the foreground figures, the drama of their activities. I am part of this picture too, that is nothing less than a masterpiece.

In this work of art there is a pervading sense of order, beauty, peace. Unobtrusively, maids come to make our beds and clean the rooms. I go out on my balcony, while they move quietly and quickly about – the only sound a soft chatter in Portuguese, and a gay acknowledgment to me as they leave. There are no vacuum cleaners, or other electrical gadgetry. They polish the corridors with great soft mops, swishing and swirling like ocean waves. Throughout the clinic there are no radios or TVs. We are restored to a world of natural and human sounds. Though the nurses and nurses' aides are dressed in crisp white uniforms, they in no way resemble their sisters in regular hospitals who tend to equate efficiency with bustling, crackling intrusiveness. Yet they are far more prompt in meeting our requests. We never have to wait, and each person gives the sense of having unlimited time. No request is too insignificant; shampoo, information on some local attraction, another cup of tea, are given the same priority as a shot of morphine in the night. And this goes for everyone: doctors, therapists, receptionists. I think the cooks would lay down their knives to attend to our needs.

The unavoidable nasty medical procedures are woven into the fabric of this healing atmosphere so that we barely notice these events. We have our blood drawn while barely awake, hearing the chink of breakfast china waiting to be brought as soon as this ordeal is complete. We have gynecological or rectal examinations gazing up at such an exquisitely painted ceiling one can almost forget the probing gloved fingers, the cold touch of the metal speculum. The X-rays and ultrasounds are conducted so swiftly, each of us called to the basement waiting rooms just before our turn, and companioned by such warmly comforting figures that any fear or discomfort is minimal. Our doctors, visiting us twice daily, combine the necessary routines and exchanges about our bodies with such a leisurely, spacious interest in the doings of our souls and spirits, that I see myself and others begin to bloom into a new sense of wholeness under their regard. The structure and rhythm of our own days is also so carefully created that we too can move through them at the same unhurried pace. Within a week I feel I have stepped into a new sense of time and space. And this outer order and harmony begins to imprint itself inwardly, fitting some long forgotten way of being like a glove to the hand.

Dr. Riggenbach has concocted a provisional package of therapies: four weekly sessions of curative eurythmy, three of water color painting, two massages and something unpronounceable which I will do at the same time every day. I raise my eyebrows at the last.
"It would be called Color-Light in English, I think," he says gravely.
"But you will soon see what it really is." He tells me there are also group eurythmy and music sessions in the early evenings which patients are encouraged to attend. I obviously can't keep the terror and dismay I feel at the thought of music out of my face, and he adds quickly: "If it's too much for you, we can always cut something out." I'll save him the trouble, and skip music I think! But I set forth for my first eurythmy session happily, and find my therapist waiting for me downstairs in the lobby in case I lose my way. She is a small, silver-haired woman with the soft skin and bright eyes of a young girl, and the peculiarly graceful movements all eurythmists seem to have. Her name is Sister Friedel. She speaks excellent English, having worked in a London hospital during the last war.

"Can you wait a moment while I fetch myself a cup of coffee?" she asks, with a twinkle. "I will have much more concentration after that." I tell her I am delighted to find that breakfast coffee is offered here. So many of the cancer diets rigorously exclude it.

"Life would be terrible without coffee, wouldn't it?" she agrees. She says she often wakes deciding they really do not need her at the Lukas Klinic, that the patients are dreadful and boring anyway and that, particularly in midwinter, she thinks it would be better if she stayed in bed. Then she makes half a cup of strong coffee, and sees immediately that the clinic is quite keen to have her services, that the patients are, in fact, very delightful and that it is worth getting dressed and walking the mile or so through ice and snow to see them all again.

While she goes off for this second cup, I find a pair of eurythmy slippers that fit and sit in her quiet rose and lilac space, smelling from across the way the delicious aromas of oils and essences that waft from the therapeutic bath and massage rooms.

We begin with Sister Friedel appraising me shrewdly, listening to what Alice already prescribed for me, pausing to gather all this into her own decision on how we might proceed. As she moves me through various exercises, forward and back, to different sounds and gestures, I can feel her process, wondering, testing out a hunch or two, as she reads my imbalances and tensions, seeking to find the particular forms and movements that may free the healing energies of my etheric body. Several times we pause, and she invites me to sit down. Though the gestures we make seems so slight, it can be tiring work. I am breathing quite heavily.

"Did you have much weight once?" she asks. "You have such broad shoulders, I wondered if you have been heavy." Except for a brief ballooning at age fifteen in Italy, and during my food research days, (neither surprising in view of the stupendous quantities of food I consumed,) I've been pretty consistently on the skinny side. I know my broad shoulders are an odd feature. Years ago someone remarked I must have been a coolie in another life. I looked as if I were still carrying that wooden yoke. I tell Sister Friedel the facts of this life and leave out the coolie fantasy. She next notes that one shoulder is higher than another, and suggests I might often carry a heavy shoulder bag. Yes, I do. She advises that I wear it a different way, slung like a school satchel around my neck. And gives me some exercises to loosen and soften the muscles around my shoulders, back and neck. At the end of our session, she comments:

"I think, with you, we will go very gentle and very slow. Just get that whole rhythmic system breathing quietly again." As I walk back to my room, very gently and slow, I feel how my breathing has quietened already. Indeed, Sister Friedel may be bringing me to a true quietness I never felt before.

I knew I would have water color prescribed for me, not clay. Frau Dr. Leroi picked out my problematic astral body on her first visit, asking me if I had bad teeth as a child. Of course I did; one glaring symptom of the erosion of life forces beginning at an early age. So I join a group of patients in the sunny basement, wondering briefly if they all have rotten teeth too.

At first I find the painting difficult. I am used to Eve, to standing way back from a large page, to bringing my whole body into a balanced uprightness. Now I sit, with a smallish square of well-soaked paper and attempt a series of exercises that I frankly don't much like. However, with the help of a student teacher, doing his practicum, I persevere. His English is limited. In fact, after a couple of sessions I question him directly. Is it possible that the only words he knows are "wonderful" and marvelous", for he is full of compliments for my watery blotches produced in these first hours. "No", he assures me. He also knows "frightful" and "terrible", but actually what I am doing appears to him as pretty good. Of course I have some experience. Many of my fellows are holding a brush for the first time. The technique of manipulating color together with a very wet page is a slow-won accomplishment. I am deeply impressed by the tremendous devotion the patients give to these sessions, and share their delight at each completed work. I watch faces grow pink, crease with little secret smiles of pleasure, as we work in unbroken silence, and realize yet again that color *is* color, and no way of confining or defining it can wholly destroy this reality.

I begin to lose myself in blue, in yellow, orange, red and green, forgetting the boundaries of the page, the people sitting either side of me, the world within or beyond this room. Once in a while, standing back at the end of an hour, I see glaringly mirrored back to me the tendencies of my own organism projected on to my paper and intimately revealed with each stroke of my brush. I am annoyed to see how little has changed in all these years, since I first depicted such things. But I carry on, pushing aside despair. Each time I leave the room, I carry the colors with me, a rainbow sap running along my veins. Like a swimmer returning to the surface after a deep dive, I can draw long breaths of cleansing oxygen, see and hear more clearly than I did before I began.

Color-Light is an eye opener in more senses than one. I even learn to pronounce the German word – *Farblichten* – but neither language adequately describes this therapy. I have no idea what to expect the first time I ascend several flights of stairs, past singing voices behind closed doors – thank God singing wasn't prescribed for me – to a little room at the top of one wing of the clinic.

A slender, gentle, middle-aged woman greets me and welcomes me into what is really no more than a tiny whitewashed cubicle. Along one side is a moulded embrasure, with a comfortable chair set facing it. The therapist explains that she will guide me through an experience of the colors, tones, vowels and crystals which "belong" to each day of the week. A sort of artistic "Wash on Mondays, Bake on Tuesdays . . ." of our English nursery rhyme. The day's color will be projected by colored light into the cubicle. Then she will play the tones of the day on her lyre. I will then speak a verse which contains the daily vowel sound and, lastly, I will handle crystals of the same color as the lights. Actually, she explains somewhat diffidently as if I might leap up off my chair at such an outlandish suggestion, we will be taking those colors, tones etc., that are created and sustained by the planet that rules each day of the week. I do not leap off my chair. Why should it not be so? I think it eminently possible that this is one of the truths we have merely forgotten. Anyway, I'm game for it.

So begins a delightful meditation in four parts. Unlike my weak attempts at inner meditation, I can readily move into contemplation of these outer sense phenomena; the vivid light which bathes me, the strange, often haunting tones that strike deep into me, the sounding forth of my own voice in a few lines of this unknown language and finally the feel and texture of a handful of quartz crystals, each containing a world of light and form. I sense my inner response to these outer impressions – a conversation that must always be going on, yet too subtle to notice, distracted as we are by our interior monologues, or our efforts to repel the louder voices of cars, telephones, radios that beset our waking days.

The most immediate and impressive response of mine in this dialogue is the creation of complementary color. After a few minutes of the colored light, the therapist turns off the switch and plunges us both into utter night. Within seconds another color appears before my eyes. This glows as vividly as the other on the screen. We both wait until I tell her it is fading away. We repeat this process three times. The after-image sometimes varies in length and intensity. I find this fascinating – and a lot of fun; two for the price of one! I also learn not to anticipate any particular shade or hue. My therapist does not. She seems interested in whatever I produce. She does tell me after a week or so that some patients who have a severely depleted immune-system produce no after-image, so this procedure is also an effective diagnostic tool. She also explains, when I question her, that it is particularly beneficial for enlivening the rhythmic system, through connecting a patient to the rhythm of the days. So it is an obvious therapy for cancers of the breast, for the chest area is the seat of the rhythmic system which is sustained by the beating rhythms of the heart and lung. Not obvious to many, I assure her, laughing. But I'm certainly grateful it became obvious to some!

Last, but not least of my individual therapies, is massage. After an appointment made on the internal telephone, I set off on another adventure to the bath and massage rooms, and wait my turn in a small room filled with the moist smells of pine, rosemary, lavender. Five minutes later I am invited into a small warm room, again restfully decorated and filled with still more delicious smells. Mr. Iseman introduces himself and, when I am undressed, covers me with a thick cotton sheet, leaving my shoulders exposed. Then he begins. Oh, what a treat this is to have the full body massage after six months of confined organ rubs. Neck, shoulders, spine, arms, thighs, calves, feet. I feel the slow gentle rhythms, first in his hands, then echoed in my own flesh; the vague tingling that heralds energies travelling freely again, as if after a long imprisonment or a long sleep. I grow warm and relaxed beneath his healing touch, burrow my face in the pillow and drift into semi-consciousness. A timeless time later, Mr. Iseman wraps me in a double layer of soft woolen blankets, and tells me to lie there resting for another half-hour. I blink up at him sleepily from my cocoon. Smiling, he points to a small clock at my side.

"This will ring," he tells me, "in case you fall asleep." Which I proceed to do promptly, the moment he leaves the room.

In fact, this whole place is sending me to sleep. At least the insomniac self who chatters, frets, makes lists, clutching at information, projects, words as if they were lifebelts to save me from drowning on the ocean of uncertainties. But such habits die hard and, inveterate conwoman that I am, I persuade myself that my motives for jerking myself awake so frequently are pure and positive. I have not just come here to be healed. I have come to learn. About myself, my condition, and about this medicine. And here are the people who know such things, who can also translate, if I wish, the esoteric language of astral and etheric bodies into the common speech of nerves, glands, hemoglobin counts. This is a golden opportunity to pick brains, increase my reservoir of knowledge and, of course, most importantly, to learn more fascinating facts about myself!

In these first days, I angle in on discussions of this kind. Why was this or the other prescribed? What underlay the various therapies? What was the state of my astral body? Why were there plump people painting and skinny ones doing clay? Despite the limitations of language, doctors and therapists seemed quite open, yet somehow our dialogues always fell a little flat. And I began to feel another stronger force at work, perhaps in me as much as in any of them. It compelled me to relinquish my need to know conceptually and begin to trust another kind of knowing, born of direct experience. I even began to be glad that language erected certain barriers and I was forced back on myself and a wordless appreciation of what was happening.

But I did not surrender too easily and with Mr. Iseman, who spoke fair English, I was still eager to discover why he might massage this, and not that. He gave brief and succinct replies.

"A lot of tension here," he said, touching my upper back though he had been spiralling his hands deliciously somewhere else. He seemed vague about whether this was a general massage, a particular one for all cancer patients, or one specifically for me.

"Rhythm, rhythm," he chanted. "That's what I give you." That was pretty obvious, so I fell silent, thinking he might prefer to speak only with his hands. And while he did so, I would feel less and less inclined to talk or think; simply to listen to his palms and fingertips. But after a while my persistent consciousness would rise again, like a bubble breaking surface on a pot of thick warm soup.

"What have you found right there?" He is working assiduously across my shoulder blades.

"That you walk with your neck," he replies, with a rich chuckle. How esoteric can you get, I think wryly, falling silent again. Let it happen, I urge myself, drifting back into the warm soup.

At one session, a visiting doctor attends. There are many visitors to the clinic; doctors, therapists, medical students, who come to observe and learn. This young woman apologizes for her cough: "It's not infectious, but I hope it won't disturb you." No, it does not. I lie, feeling the gentle rhythmic movements on my spine and neck, feel my own body, even my calves and feet begin to tingle and dance. But they talk about me, and of course I want to know what they say. When Mr. Iseman reaches my thighs he holds up a handful of flesh and displays it to the doctor with many dark, guttural "acchs" and "ichts". They do not sound like compliments and I am momentarily offended and surprised. Of all my body parts, I've felt some justifiable pride in my thighs and think they merit more positive expletives. But the "acchs" continue and I finally disentangle my face from the pillow and demand a translation.

"I don't know the English word," says Mr. Iseman. The doctor lays a comforting hand on my back.

"I have the same thing," she says. "I always thought it was normal."

"I have the same thing too," says Mr. Iseman delightedly. "None of us is normal here."

"Who *is* normal then?" I ask. Mr. Iseman thinks this is a great joke.

"Maybe nobody is normal. Nobody in the whole world." He is overwhelmed with laughter at this notion and has to suspend massage till he recovers himself.

I have to content myself with this information. Yet, with each session, I feel an image of wholeness, perhaps of "normality" guides this process and, when I empty my mind and take my attention into the fibers of my flesh, once in a while I sense this image beckoning my corded muscles and old bones. With each therapy and each day that weaves about them, I feel this image calling; out of a future none of us can know and beyond the grasp of language to describe, yet no less real because we have not yet come to it.

Chapter 21

HEALING DAYS

"Realms where the air we breathe is love,
Which in the winds and on the waves doth move,
Harmonizing this earth with what we feel above."
– Prometheus Unbound, Percy Bysshe Shelley.

The days unfold their rhythm; waking to the flute, enquiries after our wellbeing, breakfast, our doctor's visit, our injection of *Iscador*. Sister Friedel knocks gently, puts her head round the door to remind me what time my session is. Mr. Iseman calls to confirm my massage hour. We shower and dress. The mornings are spent in individual therapies, passing each other with brief greetings in the corridors. Sometimes there's space for a short walk, to post letters, or sit in a tiny park full of wild flowers and singing birds. Twice a week Dr. Leroi visits, with our own doctor and perhaps some visitors. She examines us carefully each time, refreshing her memory of each individual case. She may have a new suggestion for therapy, or a particular remedy. Therapists and doctors meet regularly as a group, together building a picture of each of us and our individual needs. She prescribes quartz oil for me to rub gently into my left breast. "Light and form," she tells me; as the quartz crystals I handle in *Farblichten* are also bringing me.

We come together at lunch. Grace, blessing, the communion feast. Our places change. We meet new people, forge deeper ties with familiar ones. We return to our rooms afterwards for the liver compress and a rest. A nurse applies a hot pad soaked in some herbal brew, then swathes our tummies tightly in soft white flannel swaddling bands; tucks us in with a hot water bottle and leaves us to sleep. An hour or so later a nurse's aide tiptoes in, bringing us crispbread and fruit tea. We are then free for the rest of the afternoon. I get up and go out. Even in rain I walk; up through the little town into the woods and hills. My favorite way is to climb the winding path through oak and beech tree, past cave and waterfall, to the little castle on the hill and sit, often alone, on the weathered stone parapet adrift with wild rose and clematis, gazing out over the valley; the small neat fields, the clustered red roofs, cows, horses, farmers tending their vines or beans and, in the distance, the great arching grey dome of the Goetheanum rising above the cherry trees.

Returning, I may stop in a little cafe. The Dom cafe is a favorite haunt of patients, behind the cathedral square. We drink mineral water, or herb teas on the little terrace, hearing only, now and again, the soft patter of passing feet or occasionally the resounding chimes of the cathedral bells. Some patients eat large slices of homemade cheesecake or rich nut and chocolate desserts. I don't know how they manage it, but such indulgences are no cause for guilt or shame. If members of the Lukas Klinic staff come by, they are likely to say they hope we are enjoying these. On my second day Marie-Thérèse advised me where I might get the best cup of coffee if I needed more than my breakfast allowance. In response to my shameful admission to Dr. Riggenbach that I still smoked the occasional cigarette, he said only: "You will see there are no ashtrays at the clinic." Another smoker told me Dr. Leroi had merely advised: "Be circumspect. And it is nicer if you do not stub them out on the grass or flowers." We must come to our choices and changes in freedom, and I notice how seldom I crave one now.

This is our time for shopping too, though I do little but look; at the exquisitely displayed jars of colored pastas, oils and vinegars full of branching herbs, the shelves of incomparable Swiss chocolates. In one tiny store, crowded with silk shirts and underwear I find boxes and bowls of crystals, and dig out a small dark heavy stone with a silvery metallic sheen. I am told it is a bloodstone, common to this area. I wonder if it is the "Soul" stone Carl Jung came from Basel to find?

At five o'clock there is group eurythmy or group music therapy. I gladly attend eurythmy, which I love to do and which is far better in a group. Many patients are mutilated and still raw from surgery; walking with difficulty or barely able to lift their arms. Others are frail, ravaged by chemotherapy or by the disease itself. Yet we gather together, stepping out gallantly to the sound of the lyre, or fragments of poems, attempting rhythms of clapping hands and marching steps that our children may have done in nursery school. We wobble, giggle, flush with delight and triumph at times, for ourselves, for each other, for the group as a whole.   And in almost every session there comes that moment when utter quietness falls as we step into the waves of that etheric ocean and are borne upon it like a fleet of well-captained ships. What a moving experience of community! We each, flushed and quietened, carry a released aura of warmth and vitality away with us as we say farewell and go our separate ways.

I had thought to skip the music therapy. Haunted by voices from my past, cruel school reports, humiliating public failures and incontrovertible evidence of my total lack of musical ability, I decided it was better not to spoil the show. But, on my second week some deeper inner wisdom impelled me to the music room, arriving late, and scuttling to an empty chair still hoping the earth might open and swallow me. The therapist – a vivacious, joyous young woman, literally glowing with warmth and enthusiasm, welcomes me gladly, apologizes that she will be speaking German, but exhorts me to enjoy myself. And so I do. In fact, as so often happens with the events we most fear, this hour turns out to be one of the happiest I spend here.

First we play instruments. Mine only has one note; I strum on a single bar of metal encased in wood with a little chamois leather gong whenever she directs me to. Others are plucking lyres, or bowing more exotic instruments. Simple enough, yet within minutes we have a full-blown orchestra. Then she invites us to sing and, though lacking German and a tuneful voice, I simply cannot resist. We are all clearly as happy as larks, singing, strumming, pounding, with rapt pink faces and bright eyes. No matter if I'm sharp or flat, I have to join this choir, and feel the angels who are surely present will forgive me if my contribution is somewhat less than heavenly. She brings the session to an end with a beautiful piece played on her own large lyre. We sit quietly as the plucked strings sound forth harmonies that pluck the strings of our own souls. Yes, we all have music somewhere in us. If we cannot get it out, at least we can let it in. I sit later on my balcony hearing still, reverberating, the tones and intervals out of which perhaps we and our world were made. As they die away, I find myself smiling too to think that a forty-year old complex can be dissolved in forty minutes – certainly quicker and cheaper than all my years of psychoanalysis!

In the lull between group therapy and supper, Dr. Riggenbach comes to call. He asks how my day has been, what I have done, suffered, enjoyed. He awaits any question or comment I have, on any subject, from particular treatments, the results of blood tests, to where I might buy a good umbrella or what to do in Basel if I'm thinking of making a trip.
"I see you're reading Parzival," he comments. "Are you enjoying it?"
"Yes. It seemed the right book to read while I was here."
"Indeed. This place is said to be one of the sites of the Holy Grail."
I *knew* it. What else could it be? This chalice set in the hills, jewelled with flowers and fruit; the trees growing with such vigor, including many that do not flourish in other valleys close by. And through all, running and tumbling, the clear sparkling streams. Here, from time to time, great violet clouds gather, spilling sudden rain, then part and pull away so that rainbows arch over the rinsed land and leaf and flower shine out vividly again. No wonder I too feel bathed in holy water, my senses rinsed clean as the land, unfurling like blossoms to receive the sound of bird and stream, the smell of turned earth, the touch of sun and wind. Senses renewed and attentive now, that need no longer shrink like a sea anenome at every whiff of danger. We live in brutal times and places, our sleep broken, our waking days afflicted by strident noises, harsh shapes and textures, synthetic colors, our air and water polluted by chemicals, our minds by unrealities – myriad attacks from within and without upon the fabric of our bodies and the fibers of our souls. Here in this sacred spot we are protected for a little while and can learn to greet the world again. "Hail", "whole" and "heal" are the words and meanings that arise from the same source and, until we can grow strong enough to carry and transform the world we know, we may need to replenish ourselves in places full

of the echoes of our forgotten divinity. I smile gratefully at Dr. Riggenbach as he makes to leave and tell him I have no further questions today.

Soon after, the gong sounds for supper and we gather again for another feast. Within a few days I am invited to join a group of friends for an evening walk that becomes a ritual until I leave. We follow the path out of town, past the watermill to the little lake. Sometimes we speak, sometimes the others talk quietly together in German and I listen with one ear to their voices, another to the rustle of small creatures in the hedgerows and the distant murmur of the waterfall. At the lake we fall silent, clustering on a wooden pier while we feed the ducks and fishes, and small birds who alight to snatch crumbs of bread provided by the clinic kitchens. A special time – of silent communion with nature and between ourselves. The great carp flicker below the water, ducks glide over the trees and skim towards the surface as if pulled by a magnet, the tall reeds rustle in the light breeze as the shadows lengthen over this tiny world of brown and green and gold. As the air cools and the dusk thickens, together, still silently, we leave and retrace our steps. How seldom people share silence, I think. And what a particular grace it is when we do.

We usually stop at a cafe on the way home. Here we chat, sipping our mineral water or *café au lait* or, for one or two, a long cold beer. Not heading up the diet sheet, but never mind! One young woman craves pizza – tomatoes certainly don't feature on our menus – but watching her eat one with such obvious relish I applaud her defection these few times. We return to the clinic before ten o'clock, whispering quietly as we wait to be let in, lest we disturb sleeping patients. A soft *"Gute nacht. Schlafen sie wohl,"* all round as we tiptoe to our rooms. This draws to a close the basic pattern of my days.

*   *   *

There are changes and disturbances. Towards the end of my first week, Frau Gantz communicates with many sad smiles that she will be changing rooms. I too feel a great wrench. Our almost wordless sharing has built a strong bond and I do not want to see her go. It appears the double room was a short term arrangement for her and she will now be moving to one with four beds. I can tell she is anxious as to who her fellows will be. Together with a nurse we carry along her things and she and I part with a warm hug. I return to the empty space and realize I am now faced with my first, perhaps only, significant choice in these weeks. I can now move into a single room myself if I want.

I do not hesitate. I go down to the office and knock on Frau Röllins' door. She welcomes me in with a cheery smile.

"I want to stay in my double room," I tell her after a few social preliminaries.

"Oh?" she looks surprised. "I thought you wanted a single one."

"Not any more. Please, can I stay?" I want this quite urgently and feel like a child begging a special treat.

"Of course, of course," she reassures me at once. "That is easily arranged. And I will change your bill." Whew! What a relief. I go back upstairs to celebrate. The room is, indeed, one of the nicest in the clinic, but I'm not certain why it mattered so much to stay in it, and I don't know who will share it with me now. Sitting in its empty tranquil space I wonder briefly if I've made a big mistake. That's not unusual. But the deed's done now and I'll have to live with the consequences. I attend my therapies, have lunch, my liver compress and rest and leave for my afternoon walk with the room still unoccupied. By this time I'm half-hoping, greedily, that no-one will arrive to take Frau Gantz's place.

When I come back from my walk I hear a murmur of voices through my door. Opening it, I see the room is full; of young people, laughing and chattering, who move aside with smiling apologies so I can meet the new patient, who is already in bed. I take in a pale, beautiful, fine-boned face, a crown of dark, Titian-tinted curls, and great, black-lashed eyes. Her mouth is parted in a small tremulous smile. In her arms lies a child; a girl about Adam's age, with blue eyes and golden hair. A sturdy fine-looking man who looks as though he spent time working outdoors, steps forward.
"Herr Egloff," he says, shaking my hand. "My wife, Frau Egloff. And," with a special smile in her direction, "our daughter, Barbara." I tell them my name and add: "I'm afraid I speak no German."
"They told us downstairs," he says. "We speak a little English. It will be good for Heidi to practise this." He and his wife smile at each other, then again at me. I only now notice her body which is so thin and frail it almost takes my breath away.
"Would you like us to leave?" asks Herr Egloff. "We are taking up your room."
"No, no. Please stay. I'm going out myself for a little while."
I leave. I go to my little park. I sit while waves of sadness and anger pour over me. "Why?" I ask. "Why? Why? Why?" I see again that crumpled heap of skin and bones, the lovely face and radiant eyes, the nestling child. Will I ever accept these things? Will this protest always rise up in me? Yesterday I sat here and wept, with gratitude for what had been given me, as the stresses dissolved in this healing environment. Now I weep for someone else, and a fate I cannot bear nor understand.

Madame Heidi (she always calls me Madame Lee) is thirty-seven. Her melanoma was diagnosed around the time that Barbara was born; first a false alarm, with a spinal tumor, then an authentic one with a tumor on her brain. She has had surgery seven times. A brain tumor was removed five days after her second child Michaël (pronounced Michayel, like the archangel) was born. She did not see him for five weeks after this. He is now two years old. She has had large sections of her interior removed. She has another tumor growing in her head. Her body looks like a badly sewn patchwork quilt, about as flat and thick, covered in rough stitches and long red scars. She came direct from hospital after six weeks there, mostly in intensive care. She barely saw her children during that time.

I learn something of this in the following days. I learn about the children. I see pictures of Michaël; a rosy, golden toddler, so delicious I want to sweep him up in my own arms. She tells me about Barbara who is, indeed, the same age as Adam, their birthdays two days apart. I learn that her husband has something to do with forest ecology. He also has an intuitive sense for healing plants which he often gathers there. Above all, I learn about Heidi, less through what she tells me, but through whom she is; a being of grace and courage, equalled but rarely surpassed by others I have known. I recall a man I knew who was dying of cancer saying to me with a vivid smile: "I'm just a walking skeleton." And I had replied with vigorous certainty: "No, Rudi – a walking spirit!" Heidi is another – though at times she can barely walk. When I think back now, that I might have changed my room, that I might not have met Heidi, I tremble at how easily this could have been. Our encounter is not one I shall easily forget.

So we both adjust to this new situation: Heidi transported from a conventional hospital into this strikingly different atmosphere, myself brought into a direct ongoing contact with someone whose sickness is more extreme than I have met, other than briefly, before. Heidi is often in great pain, and continual discomfort night and day. She seldom makes it to the dining room, having her meals on trays, but gallantly attempts a few therapies. We totter down to *Malen* (painting) together and, for a little while I think she forgets herself in swirling yellows and blues. But she often leaves before the session ends and I find her, white and exhausted, curled foetally over her wounds.

She apologizes frequently for disturbing me. But she does not disturb, as she drags herself quietly, wracked by cruel pains, to the bathroom at night, or rings for an attendant nurse. Nor does Aziz, the big North African, who comes at her call and massages her tenderly, tenderly, with his great dark hands. He tucks her round with not one hot water bottle, but two or three, stroking her bundled form till the morphine takes hold. No, I wake only because there is a thread that binds us, as we wake even before our own child has uttered a cry in the night. She disturbs because I care and am wounded by her suffering. All these months later, back in Detroit, she often summons me, a sudden tug on the thread that pulls me outside under the same stars that shine over her, calling: "Madam Heidi! How and where do you go now?" And she disturbs because it is not a simple matter of a young woman probably dying more obviously, perhaps sooner than the rest of us, but because she brings me into that place of tension between two realities: the eternal and the transitory: the fact of her immortality, so clear and shining and unchallengeable, and her mortal struggle to wrest a longer span here, with her friends and family, that she and they surely need and deserve.

* * *

So perhaps the time is here, with Madame Heidi's coming, to speak of love. I am sitting at lunch one day across from a young woman whom I've met before.

She is small, neat, wearing the wig that signals exposure to chemotherapy, with a pale drawn face and soft blue-green eyes. She makes a brave effort to eat, but clearly feels sick and looks so fragile that I feel a wind might blow her away. I know she is here because chemotherapy has been suspended. It has taken too great a toll on her. I also know she is hoping, with all this treatment, that she will not need it again. Many are here to recover their forces after conventional treatments, and many, like her, hope they need not suffer further violence to their bodies and minds. I feel a sour anger rise in me at the thought that these treatments are dignified by the name of therapy. I ask this woman how she came to the Lukas Klinic.

"My doctor sent me," she replies. Did she know about this place before?

"No. I only heard that it was very good."

"And what do you think of it now that you're here?" She looks down at her plate, then back at me, choosing her words with care. Her eyes have filled with tears. "I think," she says slowly, "that this is the first time I feel so carried by love that I can let go and be healed."

This is the moment that this truth walks through my door. What I am seeing and feeling here is love. Love in action, down to the smallest thing. And my discomfort comes from knowing how much I still have to learn. I so often think and practise love as effusive warmth and fail to see and express it in its true ways and forms. We can spill ourselves out towards others merely to experience ourselves and sometimes draw more comfort than we give. Bernie Siegel is right when he says we will come to know the power and effectiveness of love in the healing relationship. But it may only be a first step when we learn to prescribe hugs – splendid and necessary though they are – rather than doses of chemicals. No staff member of the Lukas Klinic has hugged me to date. Yet, like this woman, I feel held by deeds of love through each night and every day. It guides the quiet steps and voices of the nurses, cleaners and aides, rearranges pillows and flowers, prepares our food, tends the gardens and has fashioned these spaces with such artistic care. It waits patiently while we share our longings, our resentments, our anxieties. When Madame Heidi weeps and fumes because a friend has cut her hair too short – the last straw on the back of her sufferings – it is love that impels her doctor to put down his little tray of medicines and sit on the end of her bed, ready – so far as I can see – to listen all night if necessary. It is also love that sometimes does *not* listen to the slap and fuss of our surface ripples, but seeks to reach and hear the deeper currents sounding as they carry us where we truly long to go. Everywhere I turn I see this thing.

And I see, too, that perhaps it begins with small details, for love is born of interest, not of sympathies and desires, and it is only when we see the other – person or object – clear and whole against the sky, for what they are in themselves and not for how they gratify, that we are coming close to it. It is a committed attentiveness to what lives, grows, dies, not a vague romantic attachment to what attracts and pleases us. So we may need to start with stones, birds, blades of grass and later come to people and their complexities!

Well, I'm sure this place is not perfect. I'm sure it is full of the same struggles and weaknesses of any human community. All light throws a shadow, as there is no shadow without a light somewhere casting it. But something very fine and extraordinary is happening here. And I think it can happen because it is created by a group, not a solitary person: "When two or three are gathered together . . ." and that each function and each talent builds the whole; the maid bearing toilet rolls, the gardener trimming the hedge, the cook whipping up his exquisite confections, Dr. Riggenbach with his syringe full of *Iscador*, the lady playing her flute at dawn and, miles away – invisible and unknown, yet part of it – men hanging in oak and apple trees gathering mistletoe.

"Yes," I say to the woman, as we rise to leave the table, "I think I know what you mean."

Chapter 22

PARTINGS

"Be ready, heart, for parting, new endeavor.
Be ready bravely and without remorse
To find new light that old ties cannot give."
— Stages, Herman Hesse.

Dr. Riggenbach tells me he will not be here my final week. He's going on holiday. I feel an inner screech of protest and dismay. I look into his steady brown gaze.

"I'll miss you," I say. To my surprise, he blushes above his beard and I suddenly find myself coloring with embarrassment.

Oh, my God – how has he taken my statement? How must it be for these young doctors who do not defend themselves against personal encounter? Though they wear white coats, they do not sit behind desks, but join us at table, meet us at concerts or in the local shopping queue. They carry no armor of files and instruments to protect them from us who are so vulnerable to care and kindness and, above all, so vulnerable to the power of that archetype, the God of Healing, that stirs in the unconscious of all who seek Him, and drives us urgently to find Him working in every healer's face or hands.

When Dr. Riggenbach injected my abdomen with such careful tenderness, I felt his touch erotically, and questioned myself with shame. Have I been so untended; my body bereft of male comfort, masculine desire, that my own desire stirs as I receive the shaft of a steel syringe? Eros, too, is a dangerous god, who takes small account of the proprieties! Yet I had come to see that Eros may work in just such tender encounters between two people's flesh, and that it is often the lack of experience of love that calls its presence sexuality or desire. I know, in this moment, that the doctor who replaces Dr. Riggenbach will serve me well, and already has my trust. I also know, pure and simple, that I will miss this young man; that he as a person, and our particular relationship, is irreplaceable.

I recall our meetings; his consistent earnest attentiveness; his flashes of humor; his delicate tact, respectful heart and clear, cool mind. I recall the times I have felt, though so much younger than me, that he stood so far ahead and, quite without judgement, offered me the space to move forward into the finer person I could come to be. He would gently return those questions which were not, in fact, true questions, but merely attention-seeking statements that so many of us

129

still need to display. When I shared once that I wanted to know how to perceive the working of *Iscador* in my body, being dissatisfied with blood tests and temperature charts, he merely reminded me that following a meditative path could lead me to this perception; a focused observation of the world of nature and the being of man. And only through doing this quietly, objectively, might I truly perceive such realities, undistorted by my own predilections and needs.

He told me what I often already knew, but might not want to hear, for the cost of accepting the truth would be to develop more trust and more responsibility. Thus when I tried to needle out of him some assurance that I would not get a recurrence:

"Isn't it true, statistically, that one is more likely to have one within the first two years? And if I survive that period, it might get less likely?" He merely replied, with that direct, grave gaze of his: "If you are to have a recurrence, in two years, or in eight years, it is already being prepared in the spiritual world."

Yes, I had to grow up a bit, under the gentle guidance of Dr. Riggenbach and, uncomfortable though this has been at times, I am wishing we might have more of them. But I wish him a good vacation, and I genuinely hope he does for, as he has cared for me, I have grown to care for him independently of the impact he has had on my life.

*   *   *

Well, there are changes everywhere. At the end of each week a group of patients leave, and new ones come. A seminar is being held for medical students from Spain who fill extra tables. A charming Portuguese doctor has arrived from Lisbon, where he uses these treatments in his clinic. An Indian oncologist, Dr. Krishnamurti, who has a clinic modelled on the Lukas Klinic, is here on his sixth visit in as many years, to keep up on the latest developments. He is combining this visit with a world tour, lecturing to groups of conventional oncologists at a series of international conferences. Boston, Chicago, San Francisco are his next stops, followed by Singapore. He tells me he gives the conventional lecture, then offers time to any physicians interested in the work of anthroposophical medicine. We certainly need people like him and, indeed Dr. Leroi, with their high reputations, to build some bridges in the medical community. We so often forget we are all on the same side, fighting the same battles. Also that conventional medicine rests on as many superstitions and magical practices as its practitioners are so ready to impute to those offering alternatives.

It is an impressive testimony to the work of Dr. Leroi and her late husband who founded this clinic that it draws so many to observe and learn. I watch her sometimes; a tall, imposing figure in her seventies, with the fresh skin and bright enquiring eyes of youth, the distinctive contours of her face and body that remind me of the form and carvings of a Corinthian pillar. I wonder how she carries this work; rising at dawn to spend hours in her laboratory before visiting patients, attending work at Hiscia, where they manufacture and test the *Iscador*, travelling, lecturing, keeping abreast of everything from the latest research to my prescription of quartz oil! It is truly phenomenal and I know she must count on this team here highly. When I asked her once at lunch if we could visit Hiscia, she had arranged it within two days. I can't even remember to take my shopping list to the grocery store! I say how amazed and impressed I am to Dr. Krishnamurti, who is sitting beside me at lunch.

"Yes, yes," he says, a trifle impatiently, for my reflections have interrupted his undeniably fascinating dissertation on AIDS which is now, in some cases, being successfully treated anthroposophically, and is rampant in Hyderabad. I invite him to continue, only once interjecting a phrase about the tunnel-vision of conventional medicine which seldom sees beyond its narrow, self-selected perimeters.

"You must write," he pronounces, as we rise to leave. "Yes, yes, you must write about all this." I ask him why he should think such a thing.

"You have a way of putting things," he replies with conviction. "So that is what you must do." I am pretty amazed. So far as I am aware, in all our encounters, I've "put" less than nothing to him, in any "way" at all, being content to hear what he has to say. But he has spoken. Another person telling me this. Though I haven't put pen to paper in a couple of months, I tuck his statement away in the back of my mind, thinking that it is true that someone should write about all this, even if that someone isn't me.

*　　*　　*

The loss of several friends, and Dr. Riggenbach, by my last full weekend, is compensated by Sheila's arrival from England for four days. We were right. We can always trust our unconscious, our psyches working in tandem, to make good choices for us, whatever our minds dictate. We had said if it felt appropriate for either one of us, it would be good for both. And so it is.

She comes from Zurich where she has spent a week. She knows Switzerland and speaks German well; often travelling for Jungian conferences and meetings with old friends. She has booked into a small, local hotel, a very pleasant one, and has plenty to occupy her – visiting Basel, where Jung studied; walking, reading, planning our outings – while I do my therapies. She joins us at the clinic for several meals and is invited to participate in any of the therapies that interest her. Thus she paints, and joins our evening eurythmy group. She enjoys these, and is deeply impressed by the clinic as a whole. As who could not be?

Together, we arrange a brief, English-speaking tour of the Goetheanum. As a fairly long-term student of Anthroposophy, and member of the movement for over fifteen years, it may seem strange that I have not devoted several chapters to this building and Dornach which, after all, is the center for anthroposophical work in the world. Thousands travel here, not content until they have stood at the heart towards and from which all the blood of anthroposophical work and people flows. Not only is it my first visit to this region, but I have spent two weeks here barely glancing at the place.

There are a few reasons for this. One, I think, is that I have a heavy resistance to institutionalized movements that has probably some dark, karmic origins!

Anything that seems to set itself apart from others, from the world, is very difficult for me to enter. I may have had some nasty experiences in a monastic incarnation – or, indeed, dealt them to others! Dornach is replete with evidence of a group of people of like mind; all the distinctive features we associate with anthroposophists leap out at you the moment you cross the border from the neighbouring village of Arlesheim.

Several of us once wanted to market an "Anthroposophical Do-It-Yourself Kit": purple veils, lopsided pieces of wood, hand-beaten copper doorknobs, hand-knitted woolen stockings, a few gnomes and the inevitable black or purple beret. With this kit, one could transform any home from a decent rectangular box into a pink and purple delight, with all the corners knocked off, and sit at one's window, suitably attired, nodding sagely and spiritually at passers-by. Three steps into Dornach, and here it all is. People wear Birkenstocks, and thick wool socks, (even in midsummer.) They move slowly and meditatively with baskets of biodynamic produce on their arms, through an architectural landscape with barely a right-angle in sight. Never mind that I like and appreciate all this now and, were it not for my skinny ankles, might wear Birkenstocks myself! Never mind that I'll go a long way for a pound of biodynamic carrots, that my own house in Detroit is "veil-painted", and I search diligently in K-Mart or Kresges for pure wool or cotton underwear! I am just stuck with this dreadful antipathy to the concentrated dose. I need it diluted to digest with ease. So that is the sorry state I brought to this place.

Then, there is another side. I went twice to the Goetheanum my first week. And I did feel a deep awe, seeing this great building rising resplendently above the cherry trees. But I could not get in, beyond some antechambers housing a postcard stall and small cafe. The first time no-one spoke English at the entrance desk, and this was also the first time since I had been in Switzerland that this was so. It stunned me. People come from all over the world to visit, many hitchhiking and camping across Europe to reach this place. Many do not speak German and I wondered what impact it would have, arriving full of enthusiasm, to be rebuffed in this manner. It upset me because I do actually care a great deal for the work of Rudolf Steiner, and those who come after him; for the deep truths of anthroposophy; and for the tremendous dedication of those in Dornach and elsewhere as guardians and exemplifiers of spiritual science here and elsewhere. But, there it was – locked and unwelcoming. It was also locked the second time, but I found an English-speaking person in the postcard shop. She explained about the necessary precautions against vandalism, and I did appreciate how difficult it is to protect an historic site today. Probably all those lovely Christopher Wren churches in the City of London, in which I spent so many solitary, peaceful lunch hours, are now bolted and barred against intruders. I modified my too swift judgement, and asked her when I might get in. She said there were regular tours between 2pm and 4pm. My schedule at the clinic did not permit me to attend, so I was stumped again. Eventually, I got the number of an English-speaking guide who would take me round at my own choice of time. So Sheila and I arranged to go together and did have a delightful tour – far too brief for all that our elderly, charming and enthusiastic guide could have brought to it, but worthwhile nonetheless.

For the final reservation I felt, I am entirely to blame. I brought into this building all the images I carried of the original Goetheanum, which was destroyed by fires. I have seen many sketches and paintings of this extraordinary work: the beautiful pillars, wood carvings, paintings and colored glass; the great sculpture of the Representative of Man, depicting the Christ upright between the two great tempters, Lucifer and Ahriman – the one seducing us into the light away from the earth, the other dragging us into the material world where we forget our spiritual origins. These images left me disappointed in the present huge, spare, concrete edifice, splendid though it is, and which features, for its remarkable design and construction, in many architectural books. I could not help hankering for the first building. I guess many feel this way, and share my deep regret and horror that it was so cruelly destroyed. At least the Sculpture remains, but I thought the small chamber housing it did not do justice to its greatness, which I would have preferred to approach down some columned aisle, as one approaches the altar of a great cathedral down a long, pillared nave.

So Sheila and I pass some very special days. We walk and talk. We even nap together in hot sun, after a rich picnic at the summit of one of the highest local peaks to which we have travelled in a little bus. We go to dinner in Basel, drifting through the Botanical Gardens where, the previous week, I had gone with some of my fellow patients to see Peer Gynt. Our times together, of conversation or silence, are rare and precious, as they always are. Her visit draws to a close and, this last evening, we take our final after-supper promenade.

After a brief farewell to the little lake, we come down through the town, pausing to relish the late sun aslant the great curved roof of a farm barn, igniting rose and burnt sienna tiles till they seem afire against a backdrop of indigo cloud. We pause in the cobbled Cathedral square; silent except for the low murmur of an old couple walking home, and the softer murmur of their passing feet. From the hills bells sound; from cows and chapels, in this place of bells that Marjanna remembers as the *lietmotif* of her days hers. It is nearly three weeks since I heard a speeding car, or sniffed rank fumes of gasoline. The air here is full of the scent of cowparsley and wild rose. We come at last to a quiet green meadow, and sit attending the sunset, beginning its overture in a glory of mauve and gold.

Sheila is talking of Father, and Father images. She is describing a conference on this theme in Zurich that she recently attended; the impact it had on her. In all our years of conversations, Sheila says little that does not concern me too, though at first it may feel remote or strange. But this time I cannot grasp the "Father" bit.

I feel way out in deep field. The fatherless Parzival, water-color spreading on a wet page, rose crystals held in the hand, our voices raised in song; these fill my soul. And the knotty complexes feel distant and irrelevant.

"Maybe it's time to rescue your father from the unconscious," she's saying. "He drowned, didn't he?"

I reply, somewhat absently: "No. He was killed at sea, but buried on an island off the coast of Yugoslavia."

"I'm sorry. I always thought he drowned."

I watch the battle of light and darkness in the west; gold shot through with crimson now, the bellies of clouds a deepening purple, night curving like a great hand behind our backs, so that I feel a tingling chill from the touch of its fingers over my shoulder blades.

My mind goes suddenly quiet as land after snow. I can barely hear Sheila's footfalls as she steps gently over it. Into that white, still, silent emptiness, Alan comes; Alan, buried beneath the snows of an avalanche, here in these mountains, on my seventeenth birthday – the winter of his death casting its shadows down all these many years. I knew returning to this land would bring me full circle, for all the grieving and wondering of the times between.

"Alan," I say. Sheila nods. She knows. She has an Alan, too, who died.

I remember the two of us. I'm maybe twelve, he fourteen years old. We've gone down to play in the woods and fields of a Sussex farm, intersected by a local railway line. "Building a dam," or "looking for kingfishers", we said, to appease anxious grown-ups, who may have surmised from past experiences – Alan's hair badly singed in an attic candlelight ritual; our bloodied knees and tattered plimsolls after my underworld initiation in an abandoned tin mine – that we might be up to something wild and dangerous.

This rite of passage is, for me, the worst yet. We clamber and wriggle through the narrow pipe that carries the stream beneath the railway tracks. We must do this precisely when the train goes shrieking and fuming overhead. Alan goes first; to protect, and compel me forward. I *had* to follow where he led. The train thunders, terrible, above me. I am gasping with fright, in the dark, in the ooze and slime. I close my eyes and squiggle weakly on. When I dare open them, I see his figure silhouetted against a circle of light, beckoning me upward and out. My knight: Alan Alexander St. George, in his grubby armor of a torn shirt and grey school shorts, standing as guardian of the dark and herald to the new day.

"He was an adventurer," I say slowly. "They were all adventurers. They loved risk. And they all disappeared or died."

My father, Alan and other loves pass before my inner gaze. Sheila does not speak. The sun, in a blaze of blood and fire, slips below the trees. A cool breeze lifts over the grass. A single bell chimes nine notes.

"Perhaps now you must rescue your own sense of adventure; run *your* risks?"

We walk home in silence. I do not need to answer her. At the door we hug and part. I tiptoe past Madame Heidi and sit for a long time on my darkened balcony breathing the sweet night air. May Sarton's poem comes, unbidden, and I speak it quietly into the softly whispering trees.

> *"Without the violence, the major shift,*
> *The shudder of the earth's foundations torn,*
> *Without the great upheaval which could lift*
> *That fiery core, it would not have been born,*
> *And yet when chaos cooled, this land was here,*
> *Absolute and austere –*
> *Then, not before,*
> *It snowed.*
> *Later, by centuries and centuries,*
> *The saving water flowed,*
> *The grass arrived, dark little trees,*
> *After a terrible and rending war*
> *This land took on its fearful peace,*
> *After, and not before."*

When my tears fall, they are gentle as the last thaw before the final coming of the spring.

*   *   *

I weep once more before leaving this place. Returning to my room after lunch one day, I find Madame Heidi hunched up over her untouched place. She looks at me with great mournful eyes.
"Oh, Madam Lee, I will miss you so much."
I fly to her side. We cradle each other in our arms, rocking and sobbing out our hearts. How I will miss her too. Yet, does she know that my pain comes from knowing I take her with me – the pain of remembering? Will I ever forget her exhausted radiance as she returns from a day with her family and tells me how it felt when Michaël came rushing into her arms? Will I ever forget the morning we watched in silence the branch of a great pine tree outside our window, calculating the changing angle of light between it and a great cloud to see if the sky would clear for a fine day, and how Madame Heidi broke the silence suddenly with a small cry of anguish:
"Where is my little bird?" She had, unknown to me, watched for a particular bird each morning – a symbol of hope perhaps. How we rejoiced together when, with a flurry of wings, it appeared from nowhere to alight on that branch and cock its bright eye at us. And I saw Madame Heidi's own eyes brighten with its coming, and felt my own heart lighten as I watched her face.
I give her a little crystal: a geode, with a dark, crusted exterior and a small, jewelled cavern within. My own symbol for Madame Heidi; of her vivid spirit fashioning itself within her corroding flesh.

Dr. Schmitt, who attends us both this week, comes in as we cling together and, with one glance at us, moves tactfully to the window to give us time to pull ourselves together. "Pull ourselves together"? Perhaps we are more "ourselves" now than at many other times. At last he turns, his own eyes full of compassion.
"It is very difficult to say farewell," he comments. And I wonder how often he has seen this happen. I wonder if he knows, as I begin to know, that this is one of the truest aspects of our healing here – beginning to wake up to community, the invisible threads that bind us all?

*   *   *

I have supper on one of these last days with Jeanie Winstanley, an English curative eurythmist at the clinic; walking over to Dornach in the warm summer evening to her little apartment in the heart of this small town. Dr. Virginia Sease joins us briefly before going to give a lecture at the Goetheanum. Sitting in Jeanie's tiny, sunny kitchen, eating the delicious simple meal she has prepared, I wonder how I can feel any resistance to this place and the people with whom I can share so deeply and delightfully, and who are such outstanding exponents of anthroposophy. We laugh so much. Perhaps it is a sign of a healthy, balanced commitment to a movement or system of thought, that one is free for moments of irreverence, for being able to step outside it, and oneself, and note the comical impression we may make upon others who encounter the inevitable *persona* any movement displays? This clears a space, too, I think, for genuine and grave concerns we may have for how this work continues, how best to bring healing impulses into the world, each in our own way. We can think and believe anything we like, but, as Goethe reflected: "In the end, everything has to be done." I tell Virginia my own concern about the Goetheanum being less than welcoming to English-speaking visitors and, of course, she says she'll see what she can do.

It is, indeed hard to say good-bye, especially to those I may not meet again. I go for a last walk with my group of friends. I wish I could remember all their names. With continental formality we addressed each other by surname until, in desperation, I ask if they would simply call me Lee. But, still, I never grasped all theirs: Helga, Corinne, Pieternel – the others are lost, though their images remain. The two women from Hamburg, who looked like advertisements for health, yet had both had breast cancer the previous year. Their doctor had told them the incidence of breast cancer had dramatically increased since the Chernobyl disaster; from one in ten, to one in three! Who dares to say it is one's personal "bad karma" to get cancer? What about those who continue to build nuclear power plants? I could never exchange more than smiles with the young Swiss woman, whose sister was married to a dentist in Detroit; the language barrier was insurmountable. But I won't forget her musical voice, her graceful walk, or the way she devoured her pizza with such merry pleasure, and lingered over her cool beer! And I won't forget Pieternel, the Dutch woman, who wore clothes that instantly cheered us: sunny yellows, decorated with necklaces of exotic wooden beads. I recall one conversation I had with her when, remembering how hard I had made it for Judith – and probably many others – I asked her how it had been for her, attempting to change herself, within a circle of friends.

"Oh, my friends were only too glad to see me change," she replied with a chuckle. "I was so awful before!" I simply cannot believe that this was so; that this graceful, charming woman, with her deep wisdom and delicious humor, could have been so radically different before her illness. I can only imagine that her trials with cancer may have made her virtues even more visible.

Our last hours together are not spent in mournful contemplation of our parting. We giggle uproariously at the notion of a new community: "The Community of the Rectal Thermometer:" a worldwide network established and celebrated each time each of us – in Switzerland, Germany, France, Australia, Africa and America – retreats to the bathroom to monitor our feverish ascent after each injection of *Iscador*. Do we take our thermometers to parties? Do we retire in restaurants at the appointed hour; miss the final aria at the opera to "do our thing", while meditating on the thousands elsewhere, who may be tuning in simultaneously? In whatever way we honor our connection, I do not think it will be easily forgotten after all we've shared.

In this last week I revisit all my favorite haunts: the little castle, the little lake, the Dom Cafe, the Cathedral square. I heave slabs of chocolate, piles of bloodstones, bottles of bath oil and pounds of soft Swiss cheeses back to my room to take home to family and friends. Ruby, in the dispensary, asks, through an intermediary, if I will write a letter in English to some cousins in Ohio, and rewards me with a great vial of Rosemary Bath Milk, which I can barely fit in my bulging bags. Frau Dr. Leroi pays a last call.

"It's important that you sometimes eat something you dislike," she tells me. "That strengthens the Ego. A real act of will."

"Tapioca? Sago?" I ask, my face wrinkling in disgust. She and her team consult, seeking a translation for this abstruse substance.

"We call it Frog spawn," I say, helpfully.

"Ah! Frogs' Eyes. Yes, I know. Yes, why not? A little, now and then. Also, if you decide to do something, then do it. You must carry every intention through to the end. That is also a great strengthener."

So I really will have to write about all this! And did Dr. Leroi dash to the kitchens right after our interview to arrange for the cooks to include tapioca in our vegetable soup? For there it was, that lunchtime, a terrible slimy sediment at the bottom of my bowl. It is to her credit, or my infinite respect for her, that I managed a mouthful or two, before pushing the bowl aside!

I have final sessions with my individual therapists. Sister Friedel draws some charming diagrams to illustrate the eurythmy exercises I must continue from now on. I only hope I can imitate these successfully back in my living room in Detroit.

On an impulse, I ask her for an exercise – if there is one – that might diminish my "pre-menstrual bloat".

"Of course there is," she replies. "There's something for everything!" She gives me gestures that exactly imitate the action of the kidneys when eliminating fluid; enchanting, soft little movements that even now my kidneys are performing quietly, invisibly, in the dark caverns of my flesh.

There are gifts, too, for the nursing staff. I learn they like cakes or chocolates, and coffee, so they can celebrate together from time to time. It is with pleasure and a deep gratitude that I bring them these.

Then, as if I had not received enough, I am given a last gift myself. The message arrives that I should have two rhythmic baths before I leave. Though I half-wished I could have had these from the start, perhaps it was right that they were left to crown this experience; the icing on the cake I have devoured with such greedy pleasure over these weeks.

I go down to the steamy, sweet-smelling waiting room, and am duly summoned into the bath rooms by a pretty nurse. She invites me to choose my towel: blue or cream or rose-pink. I choose the rose. She leads me into a room in which there is a large wooden tub, the size of a rowing boat, with high sides. She helps me up a couple of steps and lowers me gently into a warm brew of water and delicious smelling milks and herbal oils. Then she begins to stir the water with her hands and arms. No machines here! No electrical jets! Just the continuing rhythmic movements she makes, dipping and turning her hands and wrists and forearms, till the water swirls in currents around my body and, as with the massage, the currents in my own flesh begin to respond. An expression of intense meditative concentration never leaves her face. My own, perhaps, echoes this. The water, gaining its own momentum, moves in great rhythmic waves up around my shoulders, back down across my abdomen and thighs. My calves, breasts, shoulder blades, tingle and fizz. After a while, she lets the currents settle and turns me over so I may receive all this again, upside down. She gives me a chin rest, so I can let myself relax utterly, without fear of drowning; so that I may, if I wish, and nearly do, fall asleep. When she has finished, she lets me lie a little longer, before helping me out and wrapping me in towels, even over my head. She leads me to a little room and helps me on to a couch. Over the towels, she shrouds me in thick wool blankets, turns out the light and invites me to sleep.

"I will wake you. Do not worry," she says, as she tiptoes quietly away. I lie in the darkness in my snug cocoon. I feel the warmth increase. I feel the waves and currents of the water echo in my body – or are they my own currents now? Are we formed out of waves of air and water, as much as waves of light and sound? I do not know. I know this is a profound moment in my life. I think of ancient rituals of initiation, and the Greek temples of healing, to which the sick and wounded were carried, and priests guided their recovery while they slept beside the central pool. I too, fall asleep, here at the heart of this temple of healing to which the grace of my destiny has led me. Without cancer, I could not have entered here!

*   *   *

The African Bushmen say you should never look over your shoulder when leaving a beloved person or place, lest you are tempted to turn back and stay for ever. I remember this as I sit, squashed between my bulging bags, in the taxi bearing me away. I face straight ahead. True, I may return one day. I may perch on the little castle walls, cradling a "soul stone" in my hands. I may meet again with some of these people, companions briefly on my journey, who are yet for all time engraved upon my heart. But now I must go forward. "Be ready, heart . . ." I murmur to myself, as the cluster of houses, the bright gardens and the blue-green hills recede.

Chapter 23

RETURN

"All things, however they flourish,
Turn and go home to the root from which they sprang."
— Tao Ti Ching.

"How old is your son?"
"I'm not going to tell you." Will she be asking this when Adam is twenty-seven, or fifty-three? "You tell *me* what you've found."
"Well, I can't see anything on your mammogram." The doctor gives me a piercing look. "But I feel in my heart that you have a recurrence." I return her gaze steadily and she has the grace to add: "Of course you know I'm expecting one."

This is the "Anniversary" of my suspicious mammogram. It is Michaelmas Day, that festival of St. Michael defeating the dragon that we celebrate to invoke our own courage to fight our battles, to find the strength to go forward into the darkness of winter, the darkness of the unknown in our lives and the life of the world. I brought more courage than I can usually muster to this appointment but, two hours and six X-rays later, it is beginning to seep away. The radiologist had returned again and again to call me back to the machine. "The doctor would like just one more." Each time the pressure intensified. Once she used a kind of spoon to capture and impale a specific area of my breast. My legs are still trembling from the pain. The pressure on my emotions has been even more acute. But I stick my ground, clutching the edge of the examining table to support myself.
"I know you are not expecting a recurrence," the doctor continues.
"Oh, no," I reply firmly. "I never said that."

For the first time since we met I have surprised, even shocked her a little, I think. And I suddenly see the gulf that separates our values and beliefs. It must be inconceivable to her that I might choose a path that offers no certainties, while she feels pledged to "save" my body at any cost. These are deep differences. Maybe she and I will never bridge them, though I hope we will one day. I can feel for her in her position, even while needing to hold my own. Beneath her undeniable commitment, both to the earliest discovery of our cancers and to directing us to treatments she considers the most secure and effective, I wonder if she may be prey to a growing wave in the collective unconscious of the medical community that I see building in power day by day. It is bearing many into an intense, at times fanatical defence of their own beliefs and procedures and I have considered that this may be because, deep down, this system knows its time is drawing to a close. "The devil fights hardest, because he knows his time is short," says Revelations. I read of doctors policing patients; of children removed from the custody of their parents who have rejected conventional treatments in favor of alternatives; of continual assaults on alternative practitioners; of increasing objections to the manufacture and distribution of natural remedies. Recently, cases have been brought against anthroposophical doctors – by state bodies or rival physicians, not by patients, who were outraged, and have begun to form organized groups to fight for the right to choose what they consider healing practices.*

We all must be aware by now that, a hundred years hence, much western "scientific" medicine will be considered utterly barbaric, based as it is on the military model of destroy, divide and conquer. Yet how tenaciously we all hold to what has given us our sense of identity before we find the courage to surrender it and plunge into the chaos and darkness that precedes the light of a new consciousness. There's too much at stake; money and power mainly, for the manufacturers of drugs and equipment particularly, to let go lightly. It's like asking the world to dismantle its war machine! But we will need to disarm it where we find it, if this planet is to survive, let alone those who inhabit it. I do understand, at least a little, of the fears that may be eating at the roots of this great "Hanging Tree". Whether or not such an awareness touches this doctor, I do not know. If it does, I can sympathize. But I cannot allow too much of it into my own life.

When I get home, I nurse my poor bruised breast. I massage it fondly with quartz oil. I even decide to inject it directly with *Iscador* for a cycle, rather than my abdomen. It may make no difference physically, but it comforts me psychologically. Actually I do wonder what the effect of six or eight doses of radiation on an extremely vulnerable area might be. Some healing systems recommend no tests or X-rays while one is in treatment as they may disturb the delicate balance in a body attempting to restore itself. I write the doctor a letter, sharing my sense that I may well pose difficulties for her, but that I need to struggle with cancer, not with members of my therapeutic team, whom I need to be open to imagining I might be healed through these various bizarre practices. She replies that she will henceforth treat me on my terms – minimum X-rays and a positive attitude! Yes, I do hope we can find some common ground, for I like and respect her enormously.

It takes me roughly a week to recover from this episode. My temperature drops dramatically and my immune-system, obviously depressed by my shaken confidence, is unable to throw off a heavy cold; my first in half a year. But, supported again by friends, by Lenny's perpetual optimism, and my own re-emerging sense of a process far greater than the simplicities (to cure or not to cure) of this disease, I recover my own vim and vigor again.

Francina tells me I am walking differently; with more rhythm and grace. A few people ask about my shoulders, which appear less hunched and tense. José

---

* *At the time of going to press, all cases appear to have been dropped.*

continues to cut my hair every three weeks and even thin it a bit. I still need long hours of sleep. Many of my bad habits are still stubbornly entrenched. It may take another lifetime to get rid of them! My eyesight has not improved, nor has my memory, despite continuing gallons of carrot juice. How did I survive those days before this mid-morning elixir? My morning eurythmy is as essential now as I always hoped meditation might come to be.

My colonics are infrequent now, since Cheri has had a baby. Though she tried for a while to make the trip from Ann Arbor, managing to deal with tubes and faucets while breast-feeding, she has cut back on her visits for a few months. I take herbal colonic rinses instead. I've lightened my intake of seeds and sprouts and *Rejuvelac*. As Mary-Jo points out it may be harder to sustain these demanding practices when one is not at death's door and can easily wonder if one has a single cancer cell. I've replaced the fever baths with swimming at the YMCA, followed by a sauna, which gets up quite a sweat. I continue to paint, and share, with Eve. We are going deeper into the whole nature of cancer now, its meaning in our times, the gift of this experience in terms of spiritual development, now that she and I are a little freer from the urgency of our personal preoccupation with our own health. I see I am only at the beginning of this journey now.

Clients return this fall, and my practice begins to fill. None have cancer! I take a wry delight in owning life's way of toppling my theories and fantasies yet again. As Steiner once said: "You may have any idea you like. Life will teach you if it's a good or bad one". Clearly a Cancer Clinic was not one of my best! Inevitably, though, I continue to meet others who have cancer and am glad to give any support I can. Suzanne's theory of women with breast cancer is that we are creating a "new sisterhood" that will flourish next time round! That's an idea that can't be toppled for a while, and I like the sound of it.

Often my gorge rises when I hear from those suffering acutely from the standard treatments, though I do own these may have saved their lives. Phyllis, who had a recurrence on her chest wall, says her doctor is treating her as if she was a house on fire. But are her charred remains, a year later, due to cancer or radiation and chemotherapy? The radiation has burned her so badly that her bones are crumbling beneath her scorched skin.
"I don't feel myself," she tells me; this woman of such imperishable spiritual vitality. Nothing has quenched her humor which I know is fashioning the world as surely as any of those lethal rays, and which will outlive her body when she decides to cast that aside.

What have my choices, my therapies brought me? When I close my eyes I am flooded with impressions, memories: *Iscador* and antimony, waves breaking at Point Pelée, a rainbow over the Jura, the loving eyes and loving touch of friends and family. The textures, tastes, smells; the gestures of beloved people; are as piercing and vivid as childhood recollections and I feel myself marvelously expanded by all the world has brought me through this year. I may not have changed that much, but I must have grown to make room in my soul for all these experiences, all these encounters.

My "Tree" has grown too; put down stronger, sturdier roots, spread its branches, sent its sap running through me night and day. Today's mail brings cards from David and Edith. David writes: "I think you've come through to some place beyond fear." No, David, but perhaps to that place of "fearful peace" that May Sarton describes. One card is a Raphael cartoon of St. Peter and St. John – faces and hands. St. Peter's eyes are full of alarm, his hands resist: "No, Lord – please not that, not there!" St. John gazes with wondering longing. His hands on his heart say: "What, Lord – me!" Is that the struggle we all face when we hear the call to tread the path onward towards our full humanity? Oh yes, there is still a long, long way to go on this sacred journey and I will need all my blood and spirit kin to accompany me. The card joins the black candle and Julian of Norwich on my mantelpiece.

A month or so after my return I learn of the death of Dr. Leroi; from a sudden massive stroke, shortly before she was due to give a conference here in America. For several nights I go out under the stars – remembering her, sending her my own feelings of gratefulness. What a gift, of providence, or my angel, that brought me to meet her in the last months of her life. I imagine the shock waves reverberating from the Lukas Klinic, throughout the world, at this tragic loss of someone so urgently needed and yet whom we must surrender to another sphere of action. So she joins John Davy, whose presence sustained me at the beginning of this thing. How comfortably sandwiched I have been between these two great souls! Another wry thought strikes me that I will now absolutely have to write. "If you have an intention, you must carry it through," were her parting words to me. Perhaps, if I persevere with this, I can leave out the Frog spawn. Tapioca and sago have not exactly headed up my grocery list!

I take the plunge and ask Dori if she will help me tease these tangled clumps of yarn into some sort of shape. She agrees, saying it will be an honor to do so, though she may find it a dubious one by the end. I'm immensely grateful for yet another talent she offers so generously to my life, as if warmth, thoughtfulness, practicality, not to mention the finest *tagliatelle al pesto* and hand-dipped chocolate cookies were not enough. I throw caution to the winds and begin to type up a storm. Whatever else, I must finish this before I die!

Not that I plan on dying yet. And I hope my sense that I still have twenty years is one life will affirm! But it is interesting to wonder what I do hope for before I reach my appointed hour.

I would like to hear a loon's cry once again. I heard my first this summer as a pair came briefly to rest on a little lake in northern Michigan. I would like to know when I was seeing my pear tree blossom for the last time. I want to see Adam move out on his own great journey into manhood and I may, if needed, compromise some of my own preferences for healing to ensure that I do. But, above, beyond, or through all this, I want to learn to know and do the "moral thing", whatever that may be at any time or place. A little more moral, anyhow! In thought, or word or deed. I do not know how to know such things, save through continual consultation with divine powers, with my own heart, and allowing others to reflect me to myself. I sense, when our lives are judged, it will not be those deeds publicly acclaimed, or even honored by ourselves that will reap reward. It will probably be a moment here or there, a word spoken or heard at the supermarket checkout, a prayer felt deeply for a fellow traveller, or a child asleep. All the unremembered moments of the heart, struggling to stretch itself a little further, till we tremor with distant earthquakes as well as for those we know and love; till we are "wise with all earth's sorrows" and its joys as well. I will need all of twenty years to learn such things, to walk a little more humanly upon this earth, but I should dearly love to take a few faltering steps before I leave it this time.

And I want more time with my friends. I am far from ready to be deprived of their glorious company!

* * *

On the Anniversary Proper of my diagnosis, we go to the farm. Rob and Mary-Jo, Karen and Paul, Adam and Matthew, to spend the day with Lulu and Al. It is a day of color, smells and tastes; bright with sun and racing clouds, a warm breeze ruffling the distant lake. We gather crimson apples, the last green beans, magenta beets, late zinnias and marigolds. We wander into the meadow bringing back armfuls of white and purple daisies, feathered grasses, branches of saffron goldenrod. Paul and Adam and Matthew throw wormy, wasp-bitten apples at the huge red barn, competing like Greek athletes. At "our age dear", I wonder, hearing Paul's shouts of glee:
"Beatcha! Didn't I? Will you *look* at that one!" Our age, or any age, – yes, why not?

Lulu and I pick salad for lunch; oak-leaf lettuce, little scarlet and golden peppers, red onions, basil, parsley, crisp snow peas. We feast on great bowls of bean soup laced with *pesto*, and local home-made pecan and apple pies. We feast on love and laughter, on Al's jokes, Lulu's embraces, little dog Ralph's contented eyes. Brimful, we walk on the beach. The grey-blue water glitters and heaves. We gather stones and shells. Each finds a silent spot, to sit with closed eyes, listening to that ancient, potent, sweetwater ocean spilling its syllables again and again against the sand. A few gulls wheel and cry. Ralph snuffles my cheek with a small, cold nose. Time to go home, she says. We call the boys who run, bringing treasures to show and share; a handmade coricle, a cluster of colored stones. We help carry them home to tea. In a crimson sunset we drive back to the city, watching the twilight deepen till the first stars prick through the blue. Does each year get better than the one before? Would these moments have half such magic if we had not struggled through to them?

A few days later, others gather round my fire. We eat brown rice and vegetables. They do not complain, though twenty years ago I had a certain reputation for *zabaglione* and glazed roast duck. We balance my ascetic offering with a rich sticky chocolate cake that Adam has made. A mutual irradiation spans the next few hours. What do we talk about? Not cancer, certainly. We cover many subjects; from the nature of the Holy Spirit to favorite recipes; how to fill in tax forms, Eastern orthodox funeral rites. Cammie describes her day at her little bookstore (Halfway-Down-the-Stairs in Rochester) which had held a little midsummer festival, the children coming through ice and snow in shorts and Hawaiian shirts to play in sand and water there all afternoon. Elaine tells us a World Conference for Colored Sheep – (lilac, pink, aqua?) – will be held this spring in Eugene, Oregon. Nancy thinks it's actually for the black sheep in our families, but I'm convinced it's the pastel shaded ones.

I confess I'm writing about this year. They are all encouraging, though Adam comments: "Who wants to know about my Mom's tits *anyway*?" Indeed! Nevertheless, we decide, since it is about all of us, we'll run the risk, forgo reticence, and jointly extend it any way we choose. Perhaps a section of "Tips for Life"? Elaine suggests Knitting for Mental Health, having read of a woman curing her agoraphobia with the comforting presence of needles and yarn. Yes, I do have a knitting pattern: "Never forget that knitting is like life itself. You will never know what shape you've made until you cast off." Perhaps I should include my recipes against anger or despair: Polishing the Kitchen Floor, Even Into the Corners; Making Three Pints of Thick White Sauce. Perhaps the world needs to know our "comforters": Fruit Smoothies, flannel nightgowns, Cornish cream teas? Reg thinks we need a section which he will submit on Clotheslines Throughout the World.

Together we agree that even a small slice of our lives could run to several volumes; perhaps compete with the latest edition of the O.E.D. which will sell at somewhere around $2,000 when complete. This is, apparently, illustrated too. There is a picture of culottes. A wise choice, Nancy thinks. One often confuses culottes with skirts. Since my sister's recently published book is called *By Way of Pain*, perhaps – suggests Nancy – we should entitle ours *By Way of Culottes*, with a cover illustration of us all wearing them? Lilac, pink, aqua? At this point Reg thinks it may be time to leave. He'll need his sleep if he is to embark on a world-wide expedition to discover foreign clotheslines. We hug each other tightly for a long, long time.

Last, but not least, I go to watch Adam asleep. Still sprawled among his furry animals. But his red pajamas have shrunk. No – his legs have grown. Long, sturdy calves protrude two or three extra inches from this time last year. How old is my son? Ten, now. And all's still well for both of us. I bend to kiss his cheek and tiptoe away, full of a deep peace and joy.

None of this, of course, will show up on my next mammogram. It will only show the slice of life I lost, but not the one I gained!

THE END

REFERENCES

Chapter 1
Carson McCullors. *Clock Without Hands.* Houghton Mifflin
Michael Crichton. *Travels.* Knopf.

Chapter 2
Deena Metzger. *Tree.* Wingbow Press.
Judith Thurman. "Spring", from *Putting My Coat On.* Covent Garden Press.
Keri Hume. *The Bone People.* Picador.

Chapter 3
Martin Buber. *I and Thou.* T.&T. Clarke.
Dr. Richard Fried, quoted in: "The Promise of Anthroposophical Medicine"
    by Richard Leviton: *East West Journal;* July 1988.
Richard Leviton. *Anthroposophic Medicine Today.* Anthroposophic Press.
Paul Pearsall. *Super-Immunity.* McGraw Hill

Chapter 4.
Dr. Rita Leroi. *Illness and Healing.* Temple Lodge Press.

Chapter 5
Eric Partidge. *Origins.* Routledge, Kegan & Paul.
Carl & Stephanie Simonton. *Getting Well Again.* Jeremy Tarcher.

Chapter 6
I Ching or Book of Changes. Routledge, Kegan & Paul
Dr. Bernie Siegel. *Love, Medicine & Miracles.* Harper & Row.

Chapter 7
Ursula Le Guin. *The Farthest Shore.* Puffin Books.

Chapter 9
Dr. Max Gerson. *A Cancer Therapy: The Results of Fifty Cases.* Worldwide
    Publishing.
Beata Bishop. *My Triumph Over Cancer.* Keats.
Dr. A. Sattilaro. *Recalled by Life.* Avon Books.
Penny Brohn. *The Bristol Programme.* Century.
Dr. G. Schmidt. *Cancer and Nutrition.* Anthroposophic Press.

Chapter 10
Hanna Kroeger. *God Helps Those Who Help Themselves.* Kroeger.

Chapter 12
Michael Ende. *The Never-Ending Story.* Doubleday.

Chapter 15
Kathleen Raine. Excerpt from "Spheres"; from *Oracle In The Heart*. Dolman
  Press.

Chapter 16
Dr. Philip Incao, quoted in: "Who Calls The Shots?" by Richard Leviton:
  East West Journal, November 1988.

Chapter 18
May Sarton. "The Silence"; from *Collected Poems*. Norton.
Philip Larkin. "I See A Girl Dragged By The Wrists"; from *The North Ship*.
  Faber & Faber.

Chapter 20
Emil Bock. *The Three Years*. Floris Books.
Rudolf Steiner. "Grace Before Meals"; from *Verses & Meditations*. Rudolf
  Steiner Press.

Chapter 22
May Sarton. "Without The Violence"; from *Collected Poems*. Norton.

Chapter 23
Sukie Colegrave. *By Way of Pain*. Park Street Press.

                        *   *   *

The Anthroposophic Society in America
National Office
529 W. Grant Place
Chicago, IL 60614

Physicians Association of Anthroposophical Medicine
P.O. Box 269
Kimberton, PA 19442

Lukas Klinic
Brachmattstrasse 19
4144 Arlesheim
Switzerland

Anthroposophic Press
RR 4, Box 94-A1
Hudson, NY 12534

                        *   *   *

Remembrance

Since completing this book, Jeanie, Sister Friedel and "Madame Heidi" – mentioned in these pages – have died. I would like to end with a loving remembrance of them, and gratitude for the ways in which they touched, and continue to touch, my life.

Order Form

Please send me _____ copy(ies) of *A Slice of Life* at $10.95 each
($13.15 Canadian). $10.95 x _____ books = _____
(Michigan Residents please add 4% sales tax.)

Shipping instructions:
I'm adding $2.00 ($3.00 Canadian) for the first copy and
50¢ for each additional copy: _____
(Allow three weeks for delivery.)

Total amount of check is: $_____

(Please make check payable to Authors' Publishing Service)

Name   _____

Address   _____

            _____

Send a copy of A Slice of Life as a gift from me to:

            _____

            _____

            _____

Published by: Distributed by:
LIFE⁄ᴇᴡᴀʏS   Authors' Publishing Services
                                    121 East Front Street, Suite 203
                                     Traverse City, Michigan 49684
                                            1-616-929-0733